Bully, Victim, or Hero?

How to Assert Yourself Without Being a Target For Bullying or Violence

Ray Amanat

DISCLAIMER

The purpose of this book is to educate. The author and/or publisher do not guarantee that anyone following these techniques, suggestions, tips, ideas, or strategies will engender success. The author and/or publisher shall have neither liability nor responsibility to anyone with respect to any loss or damage caused, or alleged to be caused, directly or indirectly by the information contained in this book.

Library of Congress Control Number: 2011933907

ISBN: 978-1-936449-06-4

Cover Design/Interior Layout: Ronda Taylor, www.taylorbydesign.com
Cover Graphics: Printing Center, LLC

References to *Tom Patire's Personal Protection Handbook* used with permission. www.TomPatire.com.

Hugo House Publishers, Ltd.
Englewood, Colorado
Austin, Texas
(877) 700-0616
www.HugoHousePublishers.com

Contents

Dedication

To my dad. You gave me my second chance at life.
I wouldn't be here if it weren't for you. I love you.

Preface

This book is designed to empower people to be heroes for themselves or others when faced with confrontations from childhood to adulthood by people who are mean or who intend to harm, otherwise known as "The Bully." It is our choice whether we decide to take the path of the Bully or the Hero.

I felt compelled to write this book because I was the victim of bullying and abuse throughout my childhood and adolescent life. I want this book to be the resource that I did not have when I was growing up. I wrote it to help present positive solutions for dealing with problems I had no answers for at that stage in my life.

This book will provoke thought for the reader and stimulate discussion between families, friends, co-workers, and the community in general. It will cover several topics from childhood to adolescence to adulthood. My story illustrates how I sabotaged myself in my childhood and adolescent years with the choices I made. I had no guidance on how to react verbally or physically in regards to the bullying and abuse. I want to explain how I turned my life around to reach my personal goals towards becoming successful in all aspects of my life.

I also want this book to bring more attention to child abuse, to bullying in schools, and to being bullied as an adult, whether it is in relationships, the workplace, or as a victim of any crime (rape, home invasion, robbery, identity theft, carjacking, etc). I went to the "School of Hard Knocks" and found out how to deal with conflict the hard way. I am sharing my experiences in this book so that you, the reader, do not have to go through what I went through growing up. Or, if you are already in a similar situation, I want to be a resource to point you in the right direction to help yourself or get help from the right people. As a child, I did not have anyone showing me positive options or positive choices so that I could successfully deal with the problems and feel safe. The decisions you make in your life when dealing with bullying or conflicts can lead you down one of two paths, one of sabotage or one of success. I would like this book to help you make better choices so you go down the path leading to success through learning how to be more assertive, rather than passive or aggressive.

I would like to thank my dad, who is my Hero and inspiration.

I also thank my brothers and my uncle for their help and support.

I thank my students, who have stuck with me and believed in me throughout my years as their mentor, especially Gail and Jary.

I thank Lisa for helping me put my thoughts on paper.

Thank you to all of the private and public schools for giving me a chance to share my experiences with faculty and students.

All of my coaches in the martial arts and my friends in law enforcement agencies and the military have been a source of inspiration to me.

These people have all been the contributing factors that have helped me find myself and the successful "third" option to bullying and violence that I present in the following pages.

Why Are You Here?

Why are you here? That is the question I ask everyone at the beginning of any lecture or seminar. I hope you are here to find a way to not be a victim of violence. But I also hope that you find out how to not being a victim to yourself based on the choices you make in your life. Because of the events from my childhood, I have chosen to dedicate my life to empowering everyone to not have a victim mindset.

So you might be reading this book because you may be in a situation where you are searching for solutions to problems and you feel you are out of options.

As a society, we have become numb to violence in the home, in our neighborhoods, in our country, and abroad. This is due in part to the bombardment of negative messages shown by the internet, the media, the music industry, advertisements, anywhere that messages are fed to us. People do not take their personal safety and well being seriously until something bad happens to them or a loved one, or something happens close to home. By letting their guard down and thinking nothing bad can happen to them, they are setting themselves up to be potential victims. As a society, we need to wake up and become "un-numbed," and be the solution that reduces the violence.

Imagine your loved one walking into the morgue to identify your body. This could be your parent identifying you, their child; your husband identifying his wife; your child identifying their parent, or any other variation. Most people will ask the question, "Why did this happen?" or "How did this happen?" I want to take you on a journey back into time and ask, "What could I have said or done differently that could have prevented this from happening in the first place?"

The military and law enforcement use the analogy that the general population is "Sheep," they are either bystanders or prey. The bully, the criminal, the terrorist, or the bad guy is the "Wolf" that preys on the Sheep. The Wolf never looks for the biggest, baddest, toughest person to pick on, confront, or victimize. They look for the weakest, meekest, shy person to torment, manipulate, and oppress; the person who does not look like they would put up a fight.

The heroes, or the protectors of the herd of sheep (law enforcement officers, soldiers, security guards, bouncers, good Samaritans, etc), are the "Sheepdogs," the ones who are trained to physically confront the Wolf, and the "Watchdogs," or those who gather information to help the Sheepdogs deal with the Wolf. For example, a small person who witnesses a crime but cannot physically help the intended target can still gather information about the criminal, like a description of the person committing the crime, their vehicle, the license plate number, etc. to pass along to law enforcement or the proper authorities. The person in the morgue is the Sheep, attacked by the Wolf. If that Sheep, or if a bystander, had been instead trained to be a Watchdog or Sheepdog, the outcome may have been different.

The problem with civilians dealing with bullies or criminals is that most have never had any type of training in threat assessment and conflict resolution. An officer goes thru the police academy and gets specialized training for dealing with different levels of threat and keeping the peace. Upon graduating from the police academy, in most cases, they are not just hired on to any law enforcement department and thrown to the wolves. They still have a support system through veteran officers, police captains, and police chiefs who show them the ropes for patrolling their territory. If the officer makes an error in judgment, they have an entire department to back them up, support them, and further educate them on how to better perform their duties. A veteran officer can take a new recruit and say, "This is how I handle these types of situations, and this is usually what I say or do to keep the peace."

The civilian generally has little or no backup. The bully, criminal, or Wolf, are always looking around to make sure that their intended target is distracted and has no other backup or a way out. The civilian, whether it is a child or an adult, may not have a support system similar to a new police officer's to give them the tools they need to maintain peace in their surroundings. If their family has never had any formal training in threat assessment or conflict resolution, how can they share any knowledge with other family members of how to handle bad situations? Law enforcement officers are trained to deal with conflict and still have a further support system for dealing with it. But there are many of us who have lived a sheltered life, never been in a fight or in any type of conflict before, and have never been shown conflict resolution. For this type of person, they only know the fight-or-flight mentality. I have worked with parents like this who have no clue about what to say or how to react in a potentially violent situation and are bringing their children to me to be their support group. I offer them something similar to what the new police officer has.

The civilian support group is made up of professionals who have dedicated their lives to educating the public in personal safety. The police officer always has some kind of backup (radios, pepper spray, taser, firearm, etc), and is trained to follow a specific protocol when dealing with conflicts. For example, the police officers' uniforms or their presence are the first stage for keeping the peace. Next are their verbal responses, knowing what to say to de-escalate a bad situation to maintain the peace or to call for backup. If the situation gets out of hand, then they use empty-handed, non-lethal use of force to detain, handcuff, and escort a subject that is disturbing the peace. If the subject resists arrest, the officer then is trained to go to the next level of force based on the guidelines of their department. Usually they will go to their pepper spray, followed by a taser gun or expandable baton, and finally, only as a last resort, their firearm.

Civilians, based on the laws in their state, do not always have all of these tools or training to aid them in dealing with any type of threat. Those civilians who do not think they have other choices or options will always resort to fight-or-flight. The people that do not want to live in fear search for alternative solutions, like purchasing a firearm or other type of device used for personal protection. Or, they seek out professionals (for example, martial arts instructors, psychiatrists, boxing coaches, firearms instructors, etc) that offer training to help build their confidence in dealing with whatever problems or issues they are going through. Through proper and sufficient training, a person can always find a way out of any type of conflict.

My goal is to train you to become a Watchdog, Sheepdog, or Hero, and not be the bystander that just watches the Hero. Imagine you were at a public swimming pool and someone was drowning. Most people would look to the lifeguard to be the hero. Some may not want to get involved for fear of lawsuits, others may not have the confidence in their abilities to help the victim, and others would assume someone else will be the one to help, and might say, "That is not my job, it is the lifeguard's job." If you were to go to a lake or a river that has fewer bystanders, more people would be apt to get involved and save the victim. If everyone were to always act as if no one else was around, and felt compelled to become the Hero in any setting, instead of being the bystander, victims would have a greater chance of survival.

My journey shows how I went from being the Sheep, or the victim, and transformed into the Wolf, or the bully, and finally made the choice to be the Sheepdog, or the Hero, someone who stands up for himself assertively. It was through training that I realized, in order for me to get the bully to leave me alone; I had to stop acting weak and meek. I had to maintain eye contact. But I also had to verbally confront the bully in a way that did not make the situation worse. I learned to use my body language to say that I was not a push-over that I would put up a fight if I needed to, in accordance with law. I eventually figured out the right equation to keep bad people on notice and away from me, yet still be approachable enough so that good people would feel comfortable around me.

My Story

Throughout my childhood, I was the victim of bullying and school violence, as well as verbal and physical abuse at home. Picture a non-verbal child in a wheelchair that has no voice to attract attention, and no use of their legs or arms to protect themselves or escape. This is how I felt when I was bullied by my peers and abused at home. I felt paralyzed. I was too afraid to run away. I did not know how to use my arms to defend myself. I did not know what to say to attract the right kind of attention for help, so I did not say anything out of fear. That is how I felt—I was literally paralyzed.

There are six main choices that most children think they have when they are put in a situation where they act out of desperation based on the environments that they grow up in. The first, if they grow up in an environment where they are exposed to drug use, they may turn to drugs. Second, if they grow up in an environment where they are exposed to alcoholism, they may turn to alcohol. Third, if their neighborhood exposes them to gang activity, they may form a new family by joining a gang. Fourth, they may run away from home. Fifth, they may become violent at home and at school. Or, sixth, they commit suicide. I was not exposed to drugs, alcohol, or gangs, so the three choices I was looking towards for myself were to run away from home, become violent, or commit suicide.

As a child, I came from a divorced family with three brothers. My parents separated when I was three years old. When my parents got divorced, the judge ruled that we could visit my dad on Wednesdays and weekends. My mom took him back to court and took away Wednesdays.

She then took him back to court again and took away Saturdays, so we were only able to be with our dad on Sundays from 7:00 a.m. to 7:00 p.m. During that time, the court systems always favored the mother more than the father, and our mother painted a very bad picture of who my father was to the court. My father fought it, but the courts favored my mother.

We were limited with the amount of contact we had with our father. The time we had with him was fun, free time, while my mother became nothing more than a bitter disciplinarian. She resented my father for his role in our lives. Because we were with our mom more than our dad, we listened to her negative messages and faced her verbal and physical abuse without knowing what to do to make things better. With our dad, we were always on our guard and did not want to bring attention to problems we were facing at our mother's home. She always said, "What happens in this house stays in this house and it is no one else's business." She intimidated us into not wanting to share anything with our father or anyone else, so out of fear we kept quiet.

When I was in school, I was the minority. My parents are both immigrants from Iran. At that time, my school was 98 percent white. I was the one who looked different. I was not the athlete or the popular kid. Everything that you can imagine that happened to a child in a bullying situation, mentally, emotionally, verbally, and physically, happened to me. At every stage, from the time I woke up to the time I got home from school, I dealt with bullies. At the bus stop, on the bus, in the hallways, in the classroom, in the bathroom, during lunch, during PE or recess, on the bus rides home. My first name is "Ray," which of course rhymes with "Gay." You can imagine the things that were said about me at that time. Because I had severe acne, the kids called me "Pizza Face." Because I am from Iranian descent, they called me "Camel Jockey, Sand Nigger, Towel Head," and other things. The school staff did not help me. Some were part of the problem. Getting off the bus, I could not just walk with friends to go to my house. From the second I got off, I would run to avoid the bullies chasing me or trying to hurt me.

In that era, most kids felt safe once they got home. (With technology today, bullying can happen 24/7 via cell phones and computers). When I got home, it was a different type of hell that I had to confront. Because of the bitter divorce from my father, my mom took out her hatred, anger, and resentment of him on my brothers and me. There was not a day when she did not let us know how much she hated our father and wished he was dead. That affected our relationship with our dad because we did not know what to believe. Our mom was a bully.

My mom was a very overprotective, controlling parent and would not allow us to do team sports for fear of us getting injured. She would hear on the news that a kid got hit by a car while riding his bike, so she would not let us ride our bikes except to the end of the driveway and back. She heard that a kid was shot at a friend's house playing with their parent's firearms, so we were not allowed to go to our friends' houses.

I was not the smartest one in the family, as my brothers were all very talented, gifted, and scholastic. I was more of the physical, motor-oriented child. So, my mom would constantly compare me to my older and younger brothers, and tell me that I was stupid, dumb, and should try to be more like my brothers. I know now that with my mom's lack of education and her upbringing that she was doing the best she could, but as a child, I did not understand this, so it did not help my situation at the time.

Between dealing with the bullying at school, and the verbal and physical abuse and fighting at home, I felt I only had those three choices: becoming violent, running away, or committing suicide. My mom brainwashed all of us into thinking our father was a bad person and someone we could not trust based on all of the negative images she portrayed of him. Since we did not have much contact with him, none of us knew what to believe.

However, out of desperation, at the age of fourteen, I took a chance and made the choice to share with my dad what was going on with me in her house and at school. I felt this was my last chance, this was it for me. I made the choice to approach my dad about not living with my mom. In my mind, if my dad would not take action and attempt to get custody of me, I would run away. If they found me and took me back to my mom, I would become violent and fight. If that did not change my mom's mind into letting me live with my dad, I would commit suicide.

My dad became my hero and took action. He took me to an attorney, who said I had to be age fifteen before I could legally decide for myself who I could live with. I was fourteen when my mom was subpoenaed to begin the process in court. When I got home from school the day she got the subpoena, it became one of the worst days of my life. She hit me and told me to call my father and say that I changed my mind, did not want to live with him, and never wanted to see him again. I locked myself in my room and stood my ground.

The more aggressive my mother became towards me, the more I knew I had made the right choice, and the more aggressive I became towards her. On another day that she slapped me in the face and, as usual, called me a "Son of a Bitch," I slapped her back, stood up and replied, "Whose son am I?" As I began standing up to her more often, she had my older brother become the disciplinarian. This became the pattern, and he and I would get into fights. I stayed with my mom close to a whole year, waiting until I turned fifteen, so I could go to court and change custody to my dad. A whole year of me sleeping with a baseball bat or tennis racket next to my bed, thinking if she hit me, I would use those to hit her back. I slept in fear and dreaded coming home from school every day, even though I could not wait to get out of school.

My relationship with my brothers and I became bitter because they blamed me for making things worse at home. I had turmoil at school, but the turmoil at home was even worse. In my mind, I said if the courts did not award custody of me to my dad, that was it for me. I would want to end it. Fortunately, the courts did award my dad custody after going through family services and counseling to make sure he could provide a safe environment for me. Their favorable reports to the court systems were what helped my dad gain custody of me.

So you can say I had a choice. To not to approach my dad and stay where I was and go down one of the six paths of self-sabotage, or take a chance and approach my dad although I did not know what the outcome would be. Because I chose to seek help from my dad, I took myself out of a negative environment where I was always being compared to my brothers, and where I hated school, made Cs, Ds, and Fs, and was constantly bullied. I moved in with my dad and became an A and B student by the time I graduated.

To illustrate a difference between my mom and my dad, when I was with my mom, I could have two Ds, two Fs, a C and a B. She would belittle me, harp on me, and ask why I had these bad grades, saying I should study more and be more like my brothers. She never praised me for any of my good grades or accomplishments. When I lived with my dad, I had those same grades, but my dad would say, "Son, I am proud of your B, and I want to see you improve on the rest," without comparing me to anyone. By focusing on my better grades, it gave me the confidence to want to improve my other grades. I became an A and B student for myself and not for anyone else.

When I moved in with my dad, I slept with the bedroom door locked because I still believed everything my mom had said about him, that he was bad and might do inappropriate things to me. This continued for a while until one day my dad confronted me about it. That is when I let him know the things my mom had said about him, and that I did not feel safe because I just did not know what to believe. My dad assured me that my mother has many issues and hatred towards him, and would say anything to make him look bad. Eventually, through seeing my dad's actions and the way that he worked with children and adults at his job, The Child Center at Our Lady of Grace, a school for emotionally disturbed children, I grew to trust my dad with everything I did and slept with the door wide open.

Now that I lived with my dad, who was not as overprotective as my mom, I wanted to do everything dangerous that you could think of that my mom would disapprove of. First, I wanted to learn martial arts, because I never wanted to be a victim of bullying or violence again. The movie *Billy Jack* and watching *Kung Fu Theater* inspired me to want to get into martial arts. I looked at several schools and came across one that I could afford and was close to my house. At the time I enrolled, the school was going through a change of ownership from one instructor to another. The new owners ran the school like the Cobra school in the original movie, *The Karate Kid.* The instructors were very aggressive, or bullies, themselves. They taught me how to be a very good bully.

I had never had an experience of what a karate school was like and thought all schools were the same. My instructors did not care for me that much at first because I was the kid that would ask all of the what-if questions. I really got on their nerves. I wanted to know everything from all points of view because I wanted to be able to handle any bad situation with confidence, and not think or react like a victim anymore, so I would constantly ask questions. I would show up every day after school, from the time they opened to the time they closed. One of my instructors admits that he purposely crossed the line with my training to try to get me to quit. However, I had one focus in mind, and that was to get my black belt and be as good of a fighter as they were. After I had trained with them for a year, and they saw that I was not going to quit, I had earned their respect. They decided that, since I was not quitting, they might as well work with me and make me the best student I could be. One of my instructors became a father figure to me, and the other like an older brother that was a drill-sergeant who always kept me in check. They both had beards, so at the age of sixteen, I had a full-grown beard and mustache, which covered up my acne. I wore nothing but black. I walked and talked like my coaches. I had become what I despised growing up, a sarcastic bully, and liked it.

At my new high school, my homeroom teacher took me under his wing and helped me feel at home in the new environment. Because I did not grow up with these kids from elementary school, I didn't have the fall-back of childhood friends. I joined the wrestling team and tried to fit in with the jocks, but that did not work, especially when they said I had to shave my beard to wrestle. That was not going to happen. I tried to fit in with the marching band, because I had started to learn to play the drums but could not read music that well, so that didn't work. I was not a bookworm like my brothers, although my grades were getting better, so I did not fit in with that clique. My friends were some neighborhood kids that went to the same school, and I wish I had taken the time to get closer to them. I had this tough-guy image in school, so people pretty much left me alone and I felt like I was just someone in the background; some of the students seemed to be afraid of me. At my old school, where I was picked on, I would walk down the hallway and avoid eye contact with everyone. Now, when I walked down the hallway, people avoided eye contact with me, and moved out of my way because I looked at them in a way that dared them to say or do anything to me. But that is the image my karate instructors developed in me. I grew my hair long, had an earring before it was popular, a beard and a mustache. My instructors introduced me to alcohol when I was seventeen years old. I just wanted to be cool and fit in by drinking and chewing tobacco. Drinking became a big problem in my life. I would come home almost every night drunk after training, and my dad told me if I did not go to AA and stop drinking, he would kick me out. Instead, I became better at hiding my habit from him. I was trying to fit in with my instructors and my peers. I did not know who I was, and tried to find myself in as many cliques as I could, but still had a difficult time finding my identity.

When I graduated from high school, I was managing the karate school and I worked as a lifeguard and assistant math tutor at the child center my dad was the medical director of. I also worked in the recreation department at a nursing home. I then decided I wanted to join the Air Force to be a fighter pilot. Because of my asthma, they rejected my application. Being immature and short-tempered, I did not think to look at other alternatives that the Air Force had to offer, so I decided to go to college for law enforcement. At that time, police officers did not have all of the computers and updated equipment they have now, nor did they have the respect of the community that they do now. So I decided not to go that route. Then I tried to start a band, but it is hard getting a group of guys together and agreeing on song lists and practice times and setting up gigs. That was too difficult to organize to make a living, so I started looking into psychology to follow in my dad's footsteps. However, I was not a fan of school and did not want to go through the many years of education that was required to get a degree.

Once I got my black belt, I decided that I was good at teaching martial arts, loved doing it, and wanted to open my own school. I had built up the school I was managing from thirty members to about eighty members. I was still training my students the way I was trained. I was the old school, aggressive, bullying instructor, and my students followed my lead and emulated my actions. At the age of twenty, my instructor suggested that I buy him out and take over the school, since I was already running the business and teaching all the classes. That is what I did.

I was twenty years old and I became a businessman. By observing the type of students I was producing, I realized that I was raising them to become everything I despised growing up, "the bully." The younger students looked up to me, walked like me, talked like me, and tried to look like me. I had a decision to make. I could continue to train my students the way I was trained, by fear and intimidation, or I could change my system and be a positive role model for my students.

I made the choice to turn my program into one where I earned my students' respect instead of me demanding it of them. I made the choice to mold my students into becoming heroes instead of bullies. I was introduced to a local D.A.R.E officer (Drug Awareness Resistance Education, through local police departments) by a personal friend. I shared with him my ideas on creating a program for teaching kids how to stand up for themselves in school without fighting. I started getting more involved with schools and the D.A.R.E. organization by sharing my program through lectures and demonstrations. It was when I began volunteering for the Special School District and Special Olympics, working with children with special needs, that I began to realize what I had, and how much I took everything for granted.

I saw and worked with kids that were non-verbal, in a wheelchair, hearing-impaired, blind, or developmentally delayed. At one end of the spectrum, there were kids that could not verbally or physically protect themselves, and were passive by nature, who were never shown how to stand up for themselves; and at the other end, kids that had either emotional or behavioral disorders, were aggressive by nature, and were in need of learning anger management and conflict-resolution skills.

These were students that could not help being the way they were. Some people looked at kids with special needs as a problem in society; I looked at them as a challenge. I wanted to come up with a program that would even out the playing field through assertiveness training by educating the passive, shy students on how to not think or react like a victim, and give the aggressive students life skills in managing their anger. Because schools have zero-tolerance or fight-free policies, I could not teach my normal curriculum of martial arts, like punching or kicking. I had to come up with a program that fit the needs of the schools in dealing with conflict resolution, anger management, and character development. My goal was to empower kids to be able to stand up for themselves without losing face in front of their peers, so they would not have to go through the things I went through growing up. As I became more involved in working with other schools, I decided to change my image.

I made the choice to stop drinking alcohol at the age of twenty-one. I did not want to be a hypocrite to my students by telling them not to drink or do drugs, and then have them see me in public somewhere drunk. I decided to cut my hair, take out the earring, and have a more professional image. I chose to change my method of teaching martial arts and my approach for educating children in the public and private school systems. I wanted to empower people of all abilities to know what to say and how to react, to help them avoid becoming victims of themselves or society, and instead become a Sheepdog or a Hero.

My training mindset went to another level. I started seeking out many different educators from different martial arts systems to come up with a well-rounded curriculum so that I could answer everyone's "what-if" questions. In the upcoming chapters, I will share how many of these mentors impacted my life and helped to shape the choices I made to become the man I am now.

Another life-altering event occurred early in my adult life. I was at home watching a "Montel Williams Show" that had caught my attention. The topic was "child abuse." The show depicted the most extreme cases of child abuse where parents would violently beat, neglect, or sexually abuse their children. They showed pictures depicting parents chaining their kids to the toilet so they could go out and party, get drugs, get out of the house and have a social life, etc. There were pictures of kids being nearly starved to death as punishment.

In one part of the segment, they had the "expert" talk about families with multiple kids. The question was brought up, "Why do the parents normally abuse only one child and not every child?" The expert's answer was that if the parents left physical signs of abuse on every child, it would bring it to the attention of neighbors, teachers, and the public much faster. When the parent singles out one child, they have the excuse of saying "my child is clumsy," or "he likes to climb trees," or "he gets hurt easily playing rough," or "he fell down the stairs" etc, which does not raise as much suspicion. As I listened and watched the segment, I was in tears. My whole childhood life with my mom flashed in front of me. Although my situation was not as extreme as those that were depicted on the show, I realized why my mom singled me out more than my other three brothers. I felt like a weight was lifted off of my shoulders, as I understood how and why my mom was who she was. The "Why Me?" question I had always had was finally answered. The program only depicted the extreme types of physical and sexual abuse and did not touch on verbal, mental, and emotional abuse like I went through, and the effects they have on children as well.

I was compelled at this point to write a letter, in tears, to the Montel Williams Show thanking them for bringing this topic to the public, and asking them to also show the other types of abuse and the effects they, too, have on children. In this letter, I expressed how I have dedicated my life towards bringing more attention to all types of violence and abuse on all levels, and how not to be the victim. Mailing this letter, even though I never got a response, gave me a sense of freedom and closure, because I finally understood my past, which helped allow me to stop living in it.

There are kids that did not have a positive parent figure or role model in their life to act as a hero and give them another choice like my father had done for me. I want to be that role model, and educate others to become role models, to let these kids know that they have positive choices they can make to have a better life.

3

Know Your Role

In understanding my past, I see that I wanted to grow up to be an adult as fast as I could, as I am sure most kids do. When I moved in with my dad, the job I had as a lifeguard at a school for troubled children put me in an adult role, as I had to be a good example to the kids that I worked with. The job I had working at a nursing home put me in an adult role caring for elders, where I was exposed to death on a regular basis. At the age of eighteen, I was managing the karate school and instructing members from ages five through adults in their sixties. Working with a wide spectrum of ages taught me how to socially communicate and forced me to grow up fast. As a teenager, I had limited guidance on the direction I needed to go towards becoming an adult. I had to figure most of it out on my own.

A big part of our culture, with technology, single-parent families, and children who do not have a strong parent figure, is flawed because somewhere we have lost the formula for taking children and mentoring them into adults. There are not many etiquette classes or "charm schools" that kids could be sent to for learning life skills. This creates a gap or a void where children look to other forms of stimulus to guide them into thinking what an adult should be. Kids are bombarded with negative messages through music, movies, books, the internet, and television. These send the wrong message about what it means to be an adult. Kids see images of sex and violence, and they fantasize about what that would be like, and try it without thinking about the repercussions or the responsibility that comes with it.

Bully, Victim, or Hero?

In our culture, adulthood is linked to sex. For boys, making it to first, second, or third base, or even home base, brings them closer to becoming an adult. For girls, they are viewed as "becoming a woman" when they get their period for the first time. This then leads to the discussion of why you have a period and what is happening to your body, which also peaks their curiosity about sex. Add this to the messages given by technology, and some feel the only rite of passage to becoming an adult is to become sexually active. The girls then become pregnant teenagers, and they both have the responsibility of parenthood at an early age.

I have found that other cultures and religions have a process that teaches children how to go from childhood to adulthood in all aspects of life. They help mold the thought process of what it means to be a father and a man, or what it means to be a mother and an independent woman, and what their responsibilities are. It teaches their role in society at each stage in their life. A child from infancy to around age seven learns that their role is to be a kid, have fun, be a sponge and be curious about the world around them, to develop social skills like sharing, taking turns, learning to communicate, and respecting elders. The role of children ages eight through eighteen is to learn responsibility, like helping around the house, doing well in school, practicing time management, learning to earn money, respecting others while earning their respect, and beginning to develop a positive value system which builds character. When children do all this, they can earn privileges, leading to more independence. Young adults are taught to know what their role is in life in order to give back to their community. The parents can guide them to become the firefighter, the mechanic, the baker, the doctor, the teacher, or the military in order to provide a service to their community or their country and give them encouragement to fulfill this role.

I have found that parents can be part of the problem when they are not involved in the growth of their child by having these discussions or activities with them. Parents have to foster and guide their kids through each phase of what is expected of them to grow into adulthood. We cannot rely on society to raise or guide our kids into knowing what adulthood is like without our influence as parents. Parents have a choice and must ask themselves if they are part of the problem or part of the solution in raising their children. The sabotage or success of the child's future begins in the parents' hands.

Parents should know their role in their child's life; and teachers, as secondary parents, should know their role as educators. A close friend and mentor, Tom Patire, a bodyguard and personal safety expert, describes this role best when teaching about parents being the protectors of their children. The parent with the most training in dealing with confrontations against the family will be the "security," verbally, and if necessary, physically, diffusing or de-escalating the situation. The parent with the least amount of training will be the "blanket" protecting the child, or their "gift." The blanket covers and evacuates the child, takes them to a pre-determined safe location, sheltering the child from being a witness to possible violence between the security and the bad guy/ Wolf. When you put both parents together, you have a "security-blanket" that protects the "gift." Sometimes a single parent has to learn to play both roles.

When our children are born, we are not given a handbook on parenting. It is through your upbringing by your parents, your values, and other resources, that you learn to become a positive role model in your child's life. Tom's program, like all things, involves time, effort, and training to understand your role. Regardless of what you are providing for your child, be it security, education, or opportunities for their growth, it is in your hands to get the training to be the best guide for your child. If your child wants you to go on a camping trip with their Scouts troop, and you know nothing about camping, it is up to you to research and learn how to camp to be a good example for your child. If your child has a discipline problem and you are having a hard time handling them, it is up to you to use all of your resources (books, social workers, the internet, etc) to find the best solutions to discipline your child in a more positive manner.

As I do presentations for schools, I share my insights as far as helping teachers know their role. It is not just the teachers' responsibilities to educate the children, but also to ensure the safety of every child. When it comes to providing a safe environment for their students, a teacher must become a Watchdog or a Sheepdog when witnessing bullying situations, or situations that become violent. For example, a small, female teacher that is around 120 pounds will not be able to break up a fight between two high- school boys that are the size of grown men. Her role as a Watchdog is to disburse the rest of the students watching, and possibly fueling the fight, to get back to class. This, in turn, helps diffuse or de-escalate the situation, enabling the School Resource Officer or other staff acting as a safety-response team, or Sheepdogs, to break up the fight and contain the situation.

In learning about my role, I personally have found that I have to go back to before I was thrown into adulthood with minimal guidance, and re-learn the things that I had not been shown as a rite to passage into becoming an adult. When I was a child, I was not given the opportunity to choose good from bad. My mother was a negative role model during my impressionable years when I should have been learning to develop responsibility as a young man. My social skills and confidence were lacking. My father was a positive role model, but it was not until I moved in with him at the age of fifteen that I was able to learn from his influence and grow and become more confident in myself.

Some people are not able to choose a positive role model from a negative role model, as both parents might be a part of the problem. So that is what they view growing up, and that is all they know. I work with people who have been through the correctional system who are trying to change their lives to keep their freedom, and their extreme stories are examples of adults who have not had the chance to choose that positive path as I did. For example, a man that has been incarcerated for being abusive to his wife may have never had a role model to show him how to be respectful to his spouse. He has to go back and review his life at the stage of learning responsibility, find what was missing from his parents (displaying love and respect, controlling anger, communicating in a healthy way, etc), and find books, articles, support groups, or counseling to re-learn healthy ways to better himself, break the negative cycle, and become a positive man.

Some of the men that I have spoken with had said that their upbringing was at one extreme where the parents were overly strict, demanding, and abusive, or at the opposite extreme where there was no discipline, guidance, or supervision. As they became adults, they said that they would not raise their children like their parents had raised them, so they moved to the opposite extreme of the way their parents were. If you are raised with one extreme, and decide to raise your family at the opposite extreme (where many people, including myself, say, "I will never raise my kids the way I was raised"), sometimes going to the opposite extreme is just as bad. For example, I was raised by an overly strict, abusive mother with lots of rules. If I, in turn, raised my child without any discipline or rules, is that really any better? It is learning to find that middle ground. So, as they become parents with kids of their own, they have the skills that are more balanced, which are needed to show their kids what it means to be a man or a woman. We all need to return to the point where our parents were no longer mentoring us in a positive manner, figure out what life lessons were missing, and choose to learn them so we can apply them to help guide us to a better path.

4

Who Are You?

"Who Are You?" was a question I struggled with throughout my adolescent and young adult life. I tried to fit in with as many different cliques as I could to try and find out who I was. I was not happy, I felt like something was missing, and had no direction as to who I wanted to become in life. I never felt right being the shy, passive Sheep, or victim. I also did not feel right being the aggressive bully, or Wolf. As an adult, I wanted to find a third option, to make sure that what happened to me in my childhood would not happen to others. In order for me to become that positive role model to help others, I knew I had to become a Sheepdog, or Hero, and make the choice and commitment to live my life as a better person.

We tend to be either passive/Sheep or aggressive/Wolf. To prove my point, I usually ask people attending my lectures that if someone were to push them or verbally abuse them, how would they react? How would you react? Generally about 80-90 percent of the responses would be to push back, hit back, or say something hurtful back, which I would call "aggressive" behavior. If you said that you would do nothing and avoid eye contact, you would more or less be like a doormat that lets people walk all over you. You would be looked at as behaving passively, and labeled as a wimp, punk, chicken, etc, and you will become the Sheep, or intended target for becoming a victim. My goal when training people is to teach them that, rather than just being passive or aggressive, there is also a third option, being assertive.

Bully, Victim, or Hero?

Here is a visual for you. If you poke a gorilla with a stick, what would the gorilla do? It would tear you apart. If you poke a lion with a stick, what would the lion do? It would eat you. If you poke a wolf with a stick, would it do? It would bite you. Humans are the only beings with the ability to be rational and reasonable. If you poke a human with a stick, they have the ability to say "Stop poking me with the stick." But, just like being pushed or called names, if the human attacks back, his behavior is like that of an animal that instinctively becomes aggressive when provoked. Normally when a wild animal attacks a human being, they are either caged or put to sleep. It is no different when a human attacks another human, they are either caged (jailed) or, depending on how severe their action, they can be "put to sleep" (the death penalty). If the human is poked with a stick and they do nothing, they are the Sheep that set themselves up for becoming the victim.

We are born with the fight or flight instinct. Assertiveness is a behavior we need to be taught in order to become rational and reasonable people. It is what separates human behavior from the animals. Government statistics say when you learn something, in order for it to become a reflex and reaction and not a thought process, you have to practice it over twenty-five thousand times. I can learn to block a punch or other type of threat, and practice it thousands of times until it becomes reflex and instinct. Before having a physical response when provoked, I have to practice verbal techniques thousands of times to make it a reflex and reaction to diffuse or de-escalate the situation so it does not go into the next phase of physical aggression. Just as I practice how to deal with physical threats in my martial arts training, I have to also learn how to deal with everyday, common threats in an assertive manner verbally, rather than immediately having an aggressive or a passive reaction. When you are trained to know how to deal with someone trying to hurt you, what does that do for your confidence and self-esteem? If you have not been trained in how to deal with this, you lack self-confidence and may become the victim.

My question at the beginning of this chapter was "Who are you?" Do you want to be the passive Sheep, the aggressive Wolf, or would you like to train to become the assertive Sheepdog or Hero? The passive, aggressive, and assertive character traits affect every role that you play in your life. I attended a conference where the keynote speaker asked the audience the question, "Who are you?" and wanted us to list as many different things to describe ourselves as we could. Right now, I would like you to take the time and make a list of all of the things that describe who you are. Do this before you read the next paragraph!

Don't cheat.

Put the book down and write your list.

Are you done yet? Quit procrastinating.

Now that I have had my fun, back to my point. I, along with most of the participants, wrote down between five to eight things that we could think of. How many did you come up with? The speaker pointed out to us that we are more than just five to eight things, and that we are limiting the way we see ourselves. Most people just list their role in the family (father, mother, wife, husband), their career, and their hobbies (a runner, a tennis player, etc). I found that there were two main categories that affect our outlook on ourselves. First, someone could list several things, but if they place no worth or value on any of these things, they see themselves as insignificant. For example, "I am just a housewife, mother, janitor, etc." Second, someone could write just one thing that they place all of their worth and values into, and neglect everything else that they are in life. For example, "I am a neurosurgeon." This person does not take into account that they are so much more to the other people in their life, like "I am a parent, I am a spouse, I am a best friend, etc." The point is to not limit our view and self-worth to only a few things, but to place value and worth on every item on your list, from the time you wake up to the time you go to sleep.

When you really break down who you are, and see all that you do for yourself and others, this helps define your character. A negative outlook of your self can also be you comparing yourself to someone else. For example, "He is a neurosurgeon, I am just a housewife." A housewife may not be saving someone's life in an operating room, but they are significant and have the responsibilities of keeping a family together and building a home based on love, care, safety, and faith.

When people asked me what I did for a living to get insight as to who I was, I would say, "I am just a karate teacher." Their reaction would normally be to take two steps back, do the Bruce Lee-scream, and take the Karate Kid stance. I could never have a serious, in-depth conversation as to what I truly do. I did not feel like people took my profession seriously. I decided to change what I told people. So I would say, "I am a teacher." They would then ask me what kind of a teacher I am. They would assume I would say a math or history teacher. When I told them I was a karate teacher, again they would take two steps back, do the Bruce Lee-scream, and take the Karate Kid stance. Finally, I realized that what I do is so much more than just teach people martial arts. I help my students develop self-confidence, well-being through fitness, a sense of safety, and a sense of purpose through reaching their goals; all of this is based on a sense of respect for themselves, their families, and others. Now, when people ask me what I do for a living, I say, "I save lives!" They ask me if I am a doctor or paramedic, and while I am neither, I *can* have a serious conversation about who I am and how I save lives.

When my eyes were opened and I saw how limited I had viewed myself, I made a new list and put down every role that I played from the time that I woke up to the time I went to bed. Now, I want you to rewrite your list, and see how much you can come up with. I have included a partial list of my own examples to help get you started:

I am a son

I am a brother

I am an uncle

I am a nephew

I am a best friend

I am a lover

I am an educator

I am a motivator

I am a boxer

I am a martial artist

I am a musician

I am a business owner

I am a consumer

I am a cook

I am a gardener

I am a motorcycle rider

I am a stepfather

I am a "chauffer" for others as a designated driver

I save lives

My dad's favorite phrase to me as I lived with him was, "*Ray, you are under-utilizing yourself.*" By looking at my current partial list, I would say that I have broken that habit. As you write your list, do not leave anything out, because everything has value. When you view yourself as insignificant, you have a tendency to not stand up for yourself, because of your lack of self-worth, which in turn can make you a victim. If, on your list, you believe you are the best at everything ("I am the s**t"), and you are full of yourself, you may be blind to the way you treat others and can be perceived as a bully. If your list shows that you are more than how you originally viewed yourself, and you feel good about who you are, you will have confidence, self-esteem, and self-worth, which leads to being assertive. When you have this sense of pride, you feel that you deserve to stand up for yourself, but in a respectful way, not in a manner that is hurtful to others. Enjoy finding out who you really are, and do not forget that everything you do has worth.

5

What Kind of a Person Are You?

Determining what kind of a person you are will give you insight on whether you are passive, aggressive, or assertive. It is ultimately your choice as to what direction you want to go with who you want to become. In order to be an assertive person, your outlook on yourself has to be one of high self-esteem, self-confidence, and self-worth. If I perceive myself as a shy introvert with low self-esteem and self-worth, I may feel that I deserve to be treated this way, and passively walk away from a fight or allow someone to continue abusive behaviors towards me. If I come across as an aggressive extrovert that is arrogant and disrespectful to others, I will not want to look small or weak in front of them, and I feel the need to save face by aggressively responding to a situation. If you have high self-esteem and self-worth, you will assertively respond to conflicts because you feel that you deserve to stand up for yourself without hurting other people, or disregarding other people's feelings. Look at who you are, and decide what your strengths and weaknesses are. You gain self-confidence by recognizing how many things you are already good at. Then, take your weak areas and slowly turn them into strengths. By doing this, you slowly build more self-esteem and self-confidence and become the assertive person you want to be, and become the hero within.

To take a better look at who you are, let's define your character. Our character is tested every day and defined by our actions based on the choices that we make. For example, the first thing a bully does in school, before picking on his intended victim, is to look around for teachers, adults, or other authority figures so they do not get caught. The first thing a criminal in your neighborhood does is to look around for police, neighbors, or the person on their front porch smoking a cigarette who may be a potential witness to their actions. They make the choice to hurt someone based on the premise that no one is watching so they will not get caught.

We all have a battle within where our good conscience and our bad conscience try to define who we are. If someone pushes you or is verbally abusive, you have the choice to either push or argue back, to avoid the conflict, or to draw attention and handle the situation in a rational manner. Your choice can sabotage you, or lead you to success. If you have peers witnessing someone pushing you, would you change your choice to not look weak in front of your peers? Do you make your choices based on peer influence or on your own?

If a person walking in front of you drops a wad of cash, and no one is around to see you pick it up, what would you do? Keep it or give it back? If there were other people around who witnessed this, would your answer change? Would your answer change if it were a lot of money or a little money? Is there a dollar level where your answer changes? Can you think of other ways our character may be tested? Now we see how much our character is tested by outside influences on a daily basis, and how that affects the choices we make. As we are faced with these outside influences, our choices help define who we want to become on the inside, or "What kind of a person am I?"

We have already made our list of who we are. Look at each item you listed, and grade yourself on what kind of a person you are based on the choices you make in that role. Grade it on a scale of one to five, one being "I am not very good at this," and five being excellent, or "this is the best I can be."

Here are my examples:

I am a son: What kind of a son am I?

Circle one   1   2   3   4   5

I am a brother: What kind of a brother am I?

    Circle one 1 2 3 4 5

I am an uncle: What kind of an uncle am I?

    Circle one 1 2 3 4 5

I am a nephew: What kind of a nephew am I?

    Circle one 1 2 3 4 5

I am a best friend: What kind of a best friend am I?

    Circle one 1 2 3 4 5

I am a lover: What kind of a lover am I?

    Circle one 1 2 3 4 5

I am an educator: What kind of an educator am I?

    Circle one 1 2 3 4 5

I am a motivator: What kind of a motivator am I?

    Circle one 1 2 3 4 5

I am a boxer: What kind of a boxer am I?

    Circle one 1 2 3 4 5

I am a martial artist: What kind of a martial artist am I?

    Circle one 1 2 3 4 5

I am a musician: What kind of a son am I?

    Circle one 1 2 3 4 5

I am a business owner: What kind of a business owner am I?

    Circle one 1 2 3 4 5

I am a consumer: What kind of a consumer am I?

    Circle one 1 2 3 4 5

I am a cook: What kind of a cook am I?

    Circle one 1 2 3 4 5

I am a gardener: What kind of a gardener am I?

    Circle one 1 2 3 4 5

I am a motorcycle rider: What kind of a motorcycle rider am I?

Circle one 1   2   3   4   5

I am a stepfather: What kind of a stepfather am I?

Circle one   1   2   3   4   5

I am a "chauffer" for others: What kind of a chauffer am I?

Circle one   1   2   3   4   5

I save lives: How do I save lives?

Circle one   1   2   3   4   5

Etc.

Now that you have completed this list, take the areas that you had low scores on (anything under three) and work on turning your weaknesses into strengths. For example, what kind of a father am I? If I am not a very good one, then what are the steps I have to take to become the father I want to be? Do I spend one-on-one time with my children? Am I involved with their school or social activities? Do I know everything I should know about who they hang out with? Am I leading by example or being a hypocrite in my child's eye? With technology today, am I guilty of ignoring my child by text messaging or talking on the cell phone, or having my child consume their free time with video games, instead of having quality time together? Am I my child's biggest influence, or is someone or something else? What kind of influence am I? Am I a hero in my child's eyes? To achieve the new and improved you, do this with each category on your list that you want to turn into your strength.

Here are a few other ways to look at who you are and how you can improve yourself. Ask yourself the following questions and see if you are surprised by your answers: How do you want people to remember you? If you meet a new acquaintance, like a potential new friend or co-worker, what would you want their first impression of you to be? What adjectives do you want people to describe you as? How would you describe yourself? What kind of impression would you want to make on a blind date? What kind of impression would you want to make at a job interview? What would you want people to say at your eulogy? What do you think people would say about you? Of course you would want to make a good impression in all categories. Sometimes we sabotage ourselves by taking our actions or our behaviors for granted. We forget that the way we behave affects others, whether the relationship is new or long-term. We only monitor our actions on the blind date, or on the job interview, where we think it "matters." We are not perfect and will make mistakes, but we should try to do our best all of the time, not just at the beginning stages of any relationship. We must all try to leave that positive, lasting impression for the people that will get to know us throughout our lives. Then, we can all be confident that the adjectives people use to describe us will coincide with those we use to describe ourselves.

One of my mentors, Mr. Joe Lewis, a former heavyweight kickboxing world champion, said it best. He explained that to become a champion, you should not put the stress of wanting to be the best in the world on your shoulders, but just focus on being the best at that moment. He tells himself, "I just have to be the best in this room!" I took that message and applied it to everything that I did from the time I woke up to the time I went to bed. For instance, you do not have to be the best father in the world, just be the best father at that moment. You do not have to strive to be the Employee of the Month, just focus on being the best employee at that moment. I did not have to be the best son in the world, I just had to be the best son at that moment. Strive to bring out your best for yourself; not for others, or for a title, or any other type of recognition.

Ask yourself this question, "Have I ever had a moment where I felt proud of an accomplishment, or did something for someone without being asked?" If you said yes, remember that feeling of pride and sense of accomplishment you had at that moment and ask yourself how it would feel to have that all of the time. The only way to replicate that feeling is to be the best at that moment. By focusing on being the best at that moment, you can only go in one direction—towards success—rather than setting yourself up for self-sabotage and potential failure.

Do You Care? If Not, Why Not?

I used to not care about what people thought about me until I saw how unproductive it made my life. I was sabotaging my own future. My dad had told me a story a long time ago about a famous guru in Iran. A wealthy man had seen this guru walking in the marketplace and said, "I am hosting a party tonight and would love to have you as a guest." The guru agreed to go to the party, which the man knew would impress all of his friends. The guru was a simple man, who was not wealthy or well dressed. When he arrived at the party, the wealthy host looked at the guru's appearance with dissatisfaction and stated, "I cannot have you here dressed like this in front of my family and friends. Here is some money, go to the market and buy some new clothes, then come back." The guru did as the host asked, bought new clothing for the party, and returned. The host, being very pleased, welcomed him in and offered him food and drink. While at the dining table, the guru took the food that was offered to him and proceeded to put it in his pockets, up his sleeves, and inside his lapel instead of eating it like everyone else. The wealthy host, confused, asked him why he was doing that. The guru replied, "You wanted me here for the clothing, not for who I am, so I felt more compelled to feed the clothing."

When my dad told me this story, I was a teenager trying to find out who I was. My interpretation of the moral of the story was to not judge others by their appearances, but also not to live your life to make everyone else happy. I used this story against my dad later on, being the rebellious son that I was. We were going to a nice dinner with some family and many of my dad's friends. I came dressed in my usual, all-black t-shirt, baggy pants, and tennis shoes. My dad said, "Ray, go put some nice clothes on before we leave for dinner." I proceeded to remind my dad of this story and asked him if he wanted me to go to the dinner for me or for my clothing. My dad did not have a reply, did not want to argue with me, and let me go dressed as I was.

Now as I look back on this, out of respect for my dad, I should have changed. While it is true that people should not judge you by your appearance, it is also true that, to be the best son I could be at that moment, I needed to respect my father's wishes due to the importance of the dinner. I was being selfish at that time, instead of selfless. Because I did not change, the dinner was awkward and uncomfortable, as I felt my father's disappointment and embarrassment, which in turn made me feel bad. I know that, if I had changed out of respect for my dad, the dinner would have been more comfortable, with the attention focused on other things besides my appearance. I failed to be the best I could be, at that moment, as a son. Who was I? I was a son. What kind of a son was I? One that did not have respect for his father's wishes. Was I being the best son I could be at that moment? No. I was a minor under the care of my father, who provided food, shelter, clothing, and other things that I could not provide for myself. I owed it to him to listen and abide by his request to show that I was becoming more responsible.

Growing up in my early childhood, I had severe acne, dandruff, and I had clothing that was outdated. I did not pay attention to my personal hygiene because I did not care due to my low self-esteem. My gym teacher in school told me in front of my classmates that I was dirty and should take more showers. My classmates, hearing this, turned it into an opportunity to bully me. As I already stated in a previous chapter, because of my Iranian descent, I have darker skin. The kids would say, "If you would take more showers, you might be white like us," on top of calling me "Pizza Face, Salt and Pepper Head," and "Sand Nigger." I had to begin to care about my appearance in order to survive the ridicule of my peers. I began to take two to three showers a day, for which my brothers nicknamed me "Shower Man," which angered my mom as well. Even though it did not stop my bullying problems at school, it did help

34

improve my self-esteem as it gave them a few less things for which to make fun of me. With every facet of your life, in growing up, if you do not care about the way people may perceive you, you may be sabotaging positive opportunities towards success with making new friends, going on a job interview, going out on a date, attending important family functions, etc.

Based on the environment that we live in, we have to make choices on how we dress and act to make the best of our situation. I was working with a student at a public school who came to class every day with his pants sagging and his underwear exposed. He would walk with a specific swagger, and talk in "ghetto slang." I asked him why he dressed, walked, and talked the way he did because I wanted to influence him and improve his appearance, like in my own personal story. His answer was not what I expected and blew me away. Most people think he dressed that way just to fit in or look cool. His response to my question was that he dressed and walked and talked that way to survive. I asked him to explain, and he said that the neighborhood that he lives in had older kids that belonged to gangs, picking on other neighborhood kids. If he were to dress with his shirt tucked in and his pants pulled up, and walk and talk appropriately, he would be singled out as a target. The older kids would think, "What are you, better than us, or smarter than us?" To avoid confrontation from the gang of kids, he said, "I just want to blend in so they would leave me alone." My comment to him was that, since he was not in the same school as the other kids in his neighborhood, he should dress and walk and talk like the person he wants to be while he is in school. But on his way home, he could dress to survive so he would not sabotage his chances for success.

The kids that do not care about anything are usually the ones with low self-esteem. I know because I was one of them. When I work with at-risk kids and ask if they care about what their parents think, or their teachers think, or their guardian thinks, their answer is, "No." I ask them if they have a role model like a sports figure or entertainer or movie star. Do they care what they would think if that figure were to walk in the room? Their answer is, usually, "No." The question is, why don't they care, and how do you get them to care? My answer is to build their self-esteem and give them a purpose or role in life. I talk to them about my experiences and how I got my self- esteem.

When I was that child growing up, I had no script and did not know what to say. I did not know how to fight, and I had a very low self-esteem. I did not care whether I lived or died. There are a lot of kids out there who have made this same equation. Not only do they not care, they are bombarded by negative messages and do not know where to go or who to turn to. The bully surgically takes away options of approaching teachers, principals, or parents to make you feel hopeless and helpless. They take away your voice. The bully will say, "What are you going to do, run to your mommy? Little mommy's boy? You gonna tell the teacher, you little tattletale?" You feel like you cannot go to your parents, teachers, or the principal, because it would make the bully right, and you want to prove them wrong. You want to stop it, but you do not know where to turn. No one is aware so no one can step up to be the Sheepdog or Hero.

What choices does that leave you, the person being bullied? Try to take matters into your own hands, become overly aggressive and build up to a Columbine situation? Run away, join a gang to have your back and make you feel safe? Commit suicide? None of these are healthy solutions to the problem because the problem still exists. If you are being bullied, and you are like me in any way, you want to be someone who could stand on your own two feet and not rely on anyone, but you do not know how.

How do you take someone that is at rock bottom, no self-esteem, no desire to live, and give them confidence and esteeming qualities to make them want to live and make something of themselves? That is the question I struggled with growing up, and that most parents ask me now when they bring their child to me to learn martial arts. All I can do is explain how martial arts or other activities, through baby steps, can change a person's life. Then I share my story with them. "Martial arts is not for everyone," I tell them. "But this is what it did for me."

I ask kids to think of something they were really proud of, a moment where they felt a sense of accomplishment. For example, winning your first trophy, getting an "A" on a difficult school project, helping the elderly or disabled, or standing up for a friend or family member. I ask them how that made them feel, and how can they build on this positive feeling.

This is exactly what martial arts has done for me as a practitioner. It is a goal-setting curriculum, where you accomplish minor goals towards the final goal of achieving your black belt. For me, someone that had no confidence and no self-esteem, the first time I broke a board made me feel like I was on cloud nine. To a lot of people, that may not be a big deal. To me, someone who did not want to live, that was a big accomplishment.

The first time I tested for my belt, from white to yellow, I had a sense of accomplishment. To some people, a yellow belt is a nobody, a beginner. You still don't know anything. But for me, not having any prior knowledge, confidence, or abilities, it was a big achievement. The first trophy I ever won at a karate tournament showed me that with training, I could accomplish greater things. A combination of many things is what gave me my self-confidence and ability to be assertive in situations. It was not just one event, it was a series of events over time that developed or shaped me from a passive, shy person into an aggressive person and, finally after realizing that there is a middle ground, the confident and assertive person. It was the journey in finding the middle ground, or the right equation, that enabled me to become assertive. With any sport or activity, you can keep trying, keep accomplishing, and get a little more fearless and have a little more sense of self-worth and confidence.

As I started performing on the demo team (we would perform at malls, boy scout camps, etc), where the audience looked at me not only as an entertainer but as someone with a special talent, I would get applause for my performances, and that built my self- esteem and improved my confidence. Every belt rank I moved up (orange, green, blue, brown, advanced browns) just kept building on and adding to my confidence, esteem, and self-worth. When my coaches entrusted me with teaching classes with lower belt students, at first it was scary but empowering. And as I have pointed out before, even though I at first used their aggressive methods in my teaching and became a bully myself for a while, eventually when I learned how to be assertive and not aggressive, it boosted my self-confidence even more.

My point is that you cannot just get a positive self-esteem or confidence in yourself overnight. It is something that builds on a series of small gains that you take and build on them. Martial arts has a curriculum that is based on achieving small goals. If you take that and apply it to anything else in your life, you can accomplish anything. I would watch the black belts, and think, "I want to be like that." Then I achieved my small goals, got better and better, and eventually I turned into the person others wanted to be like.

I became someone who has confidence, knows who they are and what they want, where they want to go with their life, and has been influenced by positive experiences and positive role models in their life. People like this will have the laser-like focus in knowing the difference between good and bad, and in being prepared by knowing how not to let the bad manipulate or control them. This takes training and guidance, and goes back to the right to passageway for that child moving into adulthood. Once I found my voice, and did not care about what the bullies thought, and communicated with my father and my teachers, I realized that I had options that the bully had robbed me of.

When I told my dad what was going on with my life with school and my mom, he gave me new options that helped build my self-esteem. He moved me in with him, got me into a new school, and allowed me to explore new activities that he did not understand but saw that they made a difference in my views for living. Martial arts allowed me to see that I was special and unique at something.

Suppose a child is constantly told that they are worthless and receives messages from their family that they are useless and will never amount to anything. Or, a spouse constantly tells you that you are worthless and do not deserve better. They belittle you, degrade you, and tell you that this is the best you will ever be. How can either ever gain any type of self-esteem? My dad told me that if I listened to the negative and became exactly what they said, I was proving them right. This is the same as the bully telling you that you are a momma's boy. Prove them wrong. If you shine a light on the problem, steps can be taken to fix the situation. Even if these steps are taken and it does not get better, when all else fails, it is your acquired confidence and self-esteem that will help you get through this and stand up for yourself.

As a parent, before your child goes away to college, you may question yourself. Have I done everything I can to show them how to survive in this world on their own? You do not have to get a black belt to learn how to protect yourself. Many parents will put their kid in a self-defense class to teach them how to survive. The parent knows they showed them how to balance a checkbook, gave them good study habits and a good work ethic, and taught them how to be polite. When you build on your child's weaknesses and turn them into strengths, you will have a sense of feeling that you have done everything that you can to prepare your child for living independently. Parents always ask themselves when the child leaves home if they have done everything. As a parent, have you done everything for your child? As a person, have you done everything for yourself to be capable of living independently without fear?

My mentor Joe Lewis taught me, "Identify your opponent's strengths and don't let him use them. Then expose your opponent's weaknesses, and use those against him." In kickboxing, your opponent may be faster than you, may be stronger than you, might have greater reach, or may be a better kicker or puncher. Once you identify what their strength is, the object is to not let them use what they are good at. Now, look for weaknesses or windows of opportunity in order to control the fight so you can win. As a fighter in a boxing ring, you become more or less a bully and turn your opponents into victims. You would literally take away your opponent's confidence and ability, and break down his self-esteem by making him feel inferior and weak. As a trainer, in order to build my athletes' confidence in their ability to win fights, I would train them as if they were my opponent, exposing their strengths and weaknesses. I would start with their strengths and build on them. I would then take their weaknesses and, one by one, give them specific drills to develop skills into making their weaknesses their strengths.

Take this training concept and apply it to the role of a parent, caregiver or educator. Anyone in a caregiver or educator's role can take a person's strength and build on it so that persons gains self-esteem. For instance, if you're a parent, when your child gets a good grade on a report or a positive remark by a teacher, praise the child for it and then encourage them to build on this success in other areas of their life: "Great job with the math grade, your hard work paid off. Let's see if you can do that with your spelling test next week also!" Then one by one, take the weak areas in their life where they lack confidence, and come up with specific "drills" to develop new skills to help take their weaknesses and develop them into new strengths, which will in turn give them a new purpose in life based on positive gains.

I posed a question to the kids during my lectures to provoke a thought process (discussed previously) that opens a discussion about self-esteem. I let them know the reason I teach is that I get a feeling of pride and accomplishment every time I see that I have made a positive difference in someone's life that I have taught. I turned my weakness into my strength. I began as the shy, introverted child that got picked on all of the time, and was afraid of speaking out, like the fighter that got his strengths and weaknesses exposed and was defeated. Then, like the fighter that was taught how to turn his weaknesses into strengths, I became someone who can now stand in front of crowds and share my life experiences with the hope that others would not have to endure what I went through growing up.

There are kids who do not have a high self-esteem or high self-confidence because they have not had enough life experiences to help them develop their personality, grow, and build their self-esteem. Ask yourself what life experiences you have had and how they have molded you into the person you are because we are all products of our environment. If the experiences that are on your list are predominately negative, is that what is causing you to make choices that sabotage your life? If the experiences on your list are predominately positive, has that lead to living a successful, happy life?

I recently worked with some boys in a juvenile detention center. I asked them to list a time when they felt proud of an accomplishment in any point in their life. Two of the boys could not come up with one example of a time when they accomplished something they were proud of. These were high school boys, and out of their entire childhood, they could not recollect one time they were proud of something they did. For these boys, not having positive experiences may have led them to commit acts that landed them in juvenile detention. If they had one positive role model, or someone to show them the ropes, who gave them the chance to feel some sense of accomplishment in any area of their life, no matter how big or small, then their outlook may have changed. They would have had one thing to feel proud of, which would lead to another thing. It helps connect the dots to look forward to other gains or accomplishments. As long as someone is praising their accomplishments, it can lead to more accomplishments.

In order to help kids develop a positive self-esteem and care about who they are and what they do, we can take something that we know they are good at in any area of their life, at home, at school, in sports, or music, and teach them to apply that confidence to everything else they may not be good at. Whether the child succeeds or fails, they learn from that experience. A true failure is someone who gives up trying. It is important to train the child to let go of their ego, which sabotages them and says they cannot do something or are not good enough. Once the ego is gone and they have developed confidence and self-esteem, our children will not be afraid to try new things, even if they risk failure at them.

When deciding on whether or not you should care, your actions and the way they impact others determine whether the outcome is positive or negative. My brother's son goes out in public wearing a superhero costume that he never wants to take off. My nephew does not care what people think, and he is not hurting anyone, so my brother allows him to do this. If my nephew wanted to wear this costume to a wedding or other important social gathering, he needs to be taught that he has a responsibility to care in this case so he does not hurt the feelings of others. The words, "I don't care" can either be used in a positive way or a negative way. You can use the words "I don't care" as long as you are not hurting yourself or others.

At the beginning of this chapter, I asked if you care, and if not, why not? When my nephew does not care and goes out in public in a superhero costume, he is not hurting anyone. But, when I did not care about what I wore when I went to dinner with my dad, I hurt him by embarrassing him in front of family and friends. As caring or not caring is like a double-edged sword, it has a dual meaning. As long as you are not hurting yourself or anyone else in any way, then you have the right to not care. Caring for yourself and others, without the ego, builds esteem and confidence in yourself and others. Make a list of all of the different ways you can show that you genuinely care for someone, without being conditional, fake, or materialistic. It is not just your words, but your actions behind the words that show you mean it.

Is It Okay to Ask for Help?

The root to most problems is your pride or your ego, not knowing how, when, where, why, or who to ask for help. A mentor and good friend, Michael Perry, said, "There is no Rambo. Every successful individual or business, including our military, is based on teamwork, which involves asking for help."

When we are at the stage of learning responsibility, from ages seven through high school, we are taught by our parents and teachers to be independent and do things on our own. For example, parents or teachers would ask, "Can you do this without my help?" When we accomplish the task, we are then praised, "Good, job, you did it all by yourself!" This is fine as long as it is communicated that, if we need help, the parents and teachers will be there to guide us. Whether it is a problem we have or a project we are working on, they try to help build our confidence and help guide us to the passage into adulthood by trying to accomplish something on our own, but also knowing that, if we need help, someone is always there to give guidance.

Some parents, teachers, or coaches try to raise the children to become Rambo's and tough guys that do not need help by saying, "Suck it up, quit being a baby, that did not hurt you, brush it off!" This trains the child to not ask for help, they feel that they just have to "suck it up." Then, if the child does have a serious problem, he does not feel he can go to the parents or teachers for help, so they are not made aware of the problem to offer a solution. The child needs guidance in learning how to do things on their own during times of difficulty, but also knowing when it is okay to ask for help when they need it. When a child is not shown this, they freeze out of not knowing what to say or do, or they make a choice that may sabotage them by getting in trouble.

If you remember from earlier chapters, when I was a child, I felt paralyzed because I did not know what to say or how to react. I did not know how to stand up for myself. The bullies at school called me a "momma's boy, teachers pet, tattletale" or "snitch," which paralyzed me and kept me from asking for help because in my mind, it would validate what they were saying and give them more reasons to tease me. Instead, I put up with the bullying, put up with the teasing, and my teachers and parents had no idea what was going on.

I also did not know where to go for help with the problems I was having at home with my mom. She had convinced me not to trust my dad, so I felt like I could not go to him for guidance. If the teachers were not aware of how to help me with the problems I was having at school, why would I think they would help me with the problems I was having at home? I was too embarrassed to speak out because I felt it would just make matters worse all around. I felt that if the kids at school found out what was going on at home, it would give them more ammunition to make fun of me.

My first martial arts instructors taught me that, if you cannot avoid the fight, start it and finish it. I felt that there was a gap or void in my training, that there was something missing in between not fighting and fighting to survive. As I was teaching martial arts, I felt that not everyone I was teaching was capable of starting and finishing the fight, so I developed four rules that I wanted all of my students to follow. The first was to try to ignore or avoid the situation. Second was to try to talk your way out of the situation, but my scripts were limited at that time. Third was to find a support group of family members, friends, or teachers. And, finally, only as a last resort, fight to protect yourself so you can get to safety. While these four rules were adequate, I felt that there was still something missing in my equation.

When I visit schools, I notice that some have students that have been raised as non-confrontational or over-protected, and would generally react by avoiding conflict or running away. Other schools, with a more aggressive student body, are more apt to hold their ground and fight. This is the fight-or-flight mindset based on their upbringing or environment. Both sides have not been taught a middle ground to save face in front of their peers and stand up for themselves without turning the situation into a violent one. This is the difference between being passive, aggressive, or assertive. We are either born passive or aggressive, but we need to be taught to be assertive.

I was at a martial arts convention and saw a demonstration by Tom Patire. I was so impressed with his program that I sought him out for training and became a certified instructor by his organization. Mr. Patire's philosophy was teaching good people to get out of bad situations. The missing element that I found from training with him was learning specific scripts of what to say and when to say them based on your age, which will diffuse or de-escalate a potentially threatening situation by drawing attention to it and attracting help from bystanders. By combining my scripts with his, I felt I could now reach and teach people on all levels and all ages more effectively. Now I had something to fill the gap, from avoiding or walking away from the confrontation, to verbally trying to diffuse it, to using fighting as a last resort. Instead of fight-or-flight, I had now found a more effective middle ground.

What are the steps for becoming assertive? What is the equation for teaching someone to be assertive when dealing with abusive or aggressive situations? For example, two kids accidentally bump into each other. One kid is aggressive and starts yelling, "Why don't you watch where you are going!" then starts provoking the second child. How would you react in this situation if you were the second person? Would you be passive or aggressive? How could you be assertive?

Below is my new list of steps to help anyone go through the progression of learning how to deal with conflict and aggression in an assertive manner, applying that middle ground.

Ray's Steps to Becoming Assertive:

Step One—Know your Safe Zone:

Many parents and teachers use the phrase "get in your personal space" or "your bubble." This, to me, is a grey area for educating or demonstrating the proper distance for feeling safe. Everybody's definition of personal space and comfort zones vary, where some people may allow others to get too close, which may place them in harm's way. If you are in a group setting with the herd, you may feel less threatened when people approach you. If you are a "stray" or isolated from everyone, your comfort zone for allowing people to get close to you needs to change. When does a bully pick on you? When you are alone. When does a criminal pick on you? When you are alone. Sometimes people that are isolated can be tricked into getting close enough where they can be hurt, or, worst case, be abducted or killed. For example, the child predator asking the child if he or she wants candy or to help find the predator's lost dog. For adults, it may be someone asking for help, for directions, for change for a dollar, or if they have a light for a cigarette. You may be distracted on a cell phone, texting or talking, which allows someone with bad intentions to get close to you without you realizing it.

Whether you are face-to-face with the bully at school or you are an adult being confronted by a criminal who is poking, pushing, and screaming at you, the untrained person will either freeze, not knowing how to react, or try to run away; the aggressive person will stand their ground and push back without backing down because of their "ego." They do not want to lose face in front of their peers. If you were face-to-face with someone and you backed down, people may consider you to be weak, a punk, a chicken, or a wimp. If the person you are facing backs down, then they are considered to be weak, the punk, the chicken, or the wimp. Because of peer pressure, both stay and the situation gradually escalates into a fight.

A "Safe Zone," by my definition, is a distance where no one can physically punch you, grab you, or kick you. A "Danger Zone" is when you are within their kicking, punching, or grabbing range. Convincing people that there is a way to step back from a confrontation without looking weak is one of the hardest things I have found to teach. We have a "safe zone," we have a "danger zone," and now we have a "comfort zone." A "comfort zone" is what type of reaction you have when confronted, which is based on how you were raised. For someone who has been raised to be non-confrontational or passive, his or her "comfort zone" would be to not fight or to run away. I have to get them to step out of their comfort zone by teaching them assertive behavior so that they learn to stand up for themselves. For someone who has been raised in a confrontational or aggressive environment, his or her "comfort zone" would be to stay, argue, and fight. They, as well, need to step out of their comfort zone and learn assertive behavior in order to not escalate the situation, which can sabotage their future.

In order for me to convince people that moving into a safe zone is the smarter thing to do, rather than staying in the danger zone to save face in front of their peers, I have to give them the following examples to make them more receptive to backing away and learn to develop a new comfort zone.

Example One: When you are in a danger zone you get tunnel vision because your focus is solely on the person in front of you, and you are not paying attention to anyone else around you. If you turn your head and look away, the "bad guy" may hit you or sucker punch you. So when I am unable to look around, I may not be aware of a second or third bad guy that may come into the picture to restrain or hold me, taking the bad situation and turning it into something worse. By staying in the danger zone, my view is also limited by not being aware of them possibly pulling out any type of a weapon, like a knife or a gun.

Example Two: I demonstrate that stepping back into a safe zone, or a distance where they cannot punch, kick, or grab me, is the smarter thing to do, because as I move away I am now able to overcome my tunnel vision and scan my surroundings. Stepping back does not mean that I am afraid or that I am a "punk." When I step back, I am able to look for exits, look for other potential threats, see if the criminal has a possible weapon, look for safe people that can get help, and look for a safe place to go. Then I am able to demonstrate that I have more time to react and more options to potentially diffuse the situation without it getting out of hand. Our goal is to find a middle ground between passive and aggressive comfort zones, and to feel good about being assertive by standing up for yourself, but still feel that you have saved face.

Step Two—Good Guy vs. Bad Guy: Reading Body Language

Your body language can either get you into trouble or keep you out of trouble. A good guy is someone who, as they step back into a safe zone, has their hands up and open in a non-aggressive, non-threatening position, which acts a barrier to protect against any strikes to the body or head. A bad guy normally has his fists up or is pointing a finger and stepping towards their intended target.

Have you ever seen this, or has this ever happened to you? Someone pushes you, and no one sees his or her action. You can choose to be passive, and be shy, avoid eye contact, and not stand up for yourself. Or, you can choose to be aggressive and push them back, where witnesses see you do it, and you are the one who gets into trouble. This may happen between siblings where they blame each other for starting it.

In other words, at one end of the spectrum, I could run away, showing passive body language and being shy or submissive. At the other end of the spectrum, I could have aggressive body language, balling up my fists or pushing back. Teaching someone to be assertive, or finding that middle ground, the "new comfort zone," is utilizing the first two stages of moving into a Safe Zone and changing your body language from being passive or aggressive to being assertive by getting your hands up and open in a non-threatening manner. With technology today, where there are video cameras all over and people can videotape with cell phones or any other personal electronic device, and because we live in a lawsuit-happy society, you never want to be perceived as the aggressor. You always want to be looked at as the person backing up and trying to avoid conflict. This, in turn, sets up Step Three.

Step Three—Stay in Control

Step Three of learning to be assertive is to keep your cool, which also means keeping your heart rate down so you can stay in control. If you let the bully or criminal push your buttons and you get angry and lose control, you are then turning control over to the bully/criminal. Do not let them control and manipulate you. Do not be aggressive, do not be passive, just keep your heart rate down by maintaining a safe distance and keep your cool. The closer you allow someone to get to you, the more your heart rate will go up, and you feel compelled to physically act out.

Your heart rate is the red flag or warning signal that is telling you to pay attention to everything around you. As your heart rate goes up, you have more of a tendency to use gross motor movements, which is the fight-or-flight response. As you keep your cool and maintain a safe distance, you are able to keep your heart rate down so you can utilize fine motor skills for maintaining control. An example of this is when an amateur boxer gets in the ring for the first time, their heart rate elevates to 120 or higher after the first round, if not sooner. At this stage, they begin to use gross motor movements, or wild punches, which exhausts them and wears them out after each round, as well as leaves openings for their opponent. If they do not pace themselves and control their heart rate and breathing, they can lose their fight. A professional boxer can go twelve rounds for a title fight and never look tired because he is able to control his heart rate and his breathing throughout his whole fight because of his practice and training.

If you have two athletes with the same skill level, weight class and size competing against each other, the first one to "run out of gas" loses. I tell my fighters "fatigue makes cowards of us all." Like the professional fighter who keeps his cool and never fights out of anger to avoid fatigue, you should keep your cool, maintain that safe distance, keep the heart rate down, and work on your breathing, so you can see more and utilize every option around you. You can apply this strategy of monitoring your heart rate to every aspect of your life (relationships, work, family, etc) as a warning sign to avoid conflict and keep it from getting out of control.

Step Four—Script for Safety

The Fourth Step is your script for safety, knowing what to say to diffuse and deescalate the situation so it doesn't get out of control. Most people have not been trained to know what to say or how to react. This is when they can lose control, so they need a script of safety to aid in attracting attention to the situation to get help or to diffuse the situation. Do not be passive and avoid eye contact, or speak in a soft-toned voice where you look weak and command no respect of anyone around you. Do not use an aggressive voice or vulgar language that would only escalate the situation to where it can get physical or out of control. The most important point of being assertive is knowing what to say to de-escalate, compromise, or diffuse a situation. Your goal is to maintain control and keep your composure. Part of learning to be assertive, and saving face in front of your peers when faced with conflict, is knowing what to say.

As we grow up, our parents give us a script for being polite, like saying "please, thank you, yes sir, no sir, yes ma'am, no ma'am." My job is to give people a script for being safe without looking passive or aggressive. The script changes for each stage from childhood, leading up to adulthood. The purpose of the script is to attract as much attention to the situation without looking like a tattletale or a snitch, with the hope that there will be a Watchdog or a Sheepdog there to help bail you out.

To help kids understand the difference between tattling and reporting something bad, I role play the following scenarios with them: If Bobby pushes me, and I go to the teacher and say, "Teacher, Bobby keeps pushing me," most people would say that I am a whining, crybaby tattletale. Now, if Bobby pushed me and I were to just move back into a safe zone, get my hands up in a good-guy position, and in a medium to loud voice, say, "Bobby STOP pushing me!" I get the attention of other students and possibly the teacher. Now I am viewed not as someone who is tattling, but someone who is standing up for himself by bringing attention to the situation at hand.

In training the bystanders to be a part of the solution and not the problem, I include them in that same role-play. As Bobby pushes me, I go through my stages of moving into a safe zone, getting my hands up into a good guy stance, keeping my cool, and attracting attention by saying "Stop pushing me, Bobby!" Melissa, the bystander, gets a teacher and informs her that Bobby is hurting Ray. Most people would say that Melissa is being a tattletale or a snitch. I say that Melissa is being a Hero. I use the example that if a house were on fire with people inside it, and Melissa calls 911, as the fire department, police, ambulance, and eventually the media come, they save the family and view Melissa as the person who helped save the day. By calling 911, was she being a tattletale or was she being a Hero? It involved saving a family from being hurt, which is no different from her reporting something bad that happened at school between Bobby and Ray, which involves saving Ray from being hurt.

Getting people to realize that using their words, or script, and saying the right things to attract attention to get help, is a hard sell. I have to visually demonstrate the importance of using that script of safety. In my lectures, I usually bring a volunteer from the audience that is considerably bigger than me. They have all the advantages of size, reach, and strength. I introduce to the audience that the only way that I can win in a conflict with this larger person, if I have no formal training, is by attracting attention to the situation. I demonstrate how a script can work and show everyone how many sheepdogs there are out there that are willing to help if you say the right thing to attract them.

Bully, Victim, or Hero?

Below you will find a dot, which represents *you*. Each diagram will show how your Network, or people who are there to help, expands. I will relate this to a child in school at first, and then show you how to use it as an adult. At school, the first responder that is a responsible adult to help a child is usually a teacher.

If the teacher needs help, they usually call the office to get the principal.

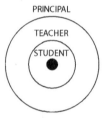

If the situation is so out of control that the principal and teacher need help, schools usually go into lockdown and a School Resource Officer ("SRO") or a response team runs to help diffuse the situation.

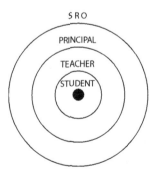

If the situation is similar to a Virginia Tech scenario, law enforcement is then called.

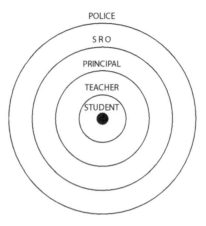

If the police need help in containing the situation, usually for worst-case scenarios like bomb threats or a Columbine-type situation with multiple shooters, the specialty teams of SWAT or Bomb Squad are brought in.

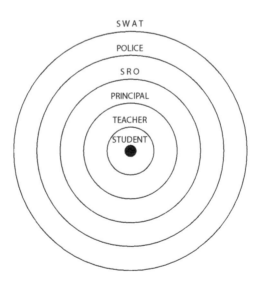

SWAT or Bomb Squad is then followed by the FBI.

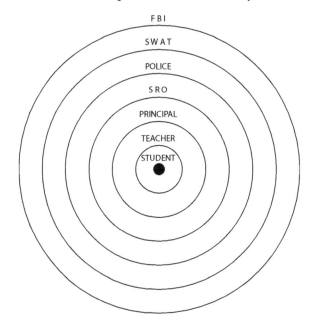

In extreme situations, the National Guard is called.

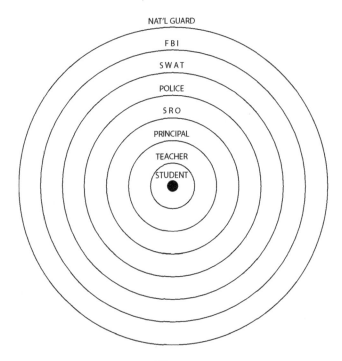

When a smaller student realizes that they can attract that much attention using their words or script in an assertive manner loudly enough to get a teacher's attention when confronted by the bigger bully, they then have the confidence of knowing that a whole network of people is at their fingertips to help. This, in turn, makes the bully look small and helps build the confidence of the intended victim.

This network of safety travels with you everywhere you go. For example, if I were at a restaurant, and I was being confronted by someone aggressively, my first responder would be my waitress, who in turn gets the manager, who calls the police, and in worst-case scenarios, SWAT, FBI, and National Guard. It is knowing the right thing to say to attract the right kind of attention.

Kids may be reluctant to ask for help because of their "egos," as they do not want to look weak in front of their peers. One way I use to convince kids in school to use their words to attract attention to get help is by proving to them that they will all eventually turn into tattletales or snitches when they become adults. Most of the kids will roll their eyes and exclaim, "No way, nuh-uh! Not me!" So, this is what I do. I bring up a teacher or adult and ask them what they would do if I were to spray paint their car pink, yellow, and bright green. Their response is usually, "I would call the police." So I say, "So you will be a snitch by calling the police to get me in trouble." I ask the kids what they would do if it was their car, and I get answers like, "I would beat you up, I would hit you with a baseball bat, I would run over you with my car." All of these would sabotage them by getting them in trouble. Most kids do not think twice about doing something extreme because they have fewer responsibilities than an adult. They may think that the only consequence of getting in trouble is getting suspended or expelled. They think "yeah, no school for a few days." At worse, they get sent to juvenile detention, where they just get a slap on the wrist, but they know mommy and daddy will bail them out. In other words, they do not have much to lose. The more the child feels they have nothing to lose by getting in trouble, knowing that their parents will bail them out, the more they will choose to sabotage themselves by behaving inappropriately.

The adult who calls the police thinks twice about taking physical action because they have more responsibilities and more to lose. If the adult were to take matters into their own hands and physically hurt the person who spray-painted their car, they stand to lose their car, their house, their family, and their freedom if they get put in jail. Your network of safety is all of the resources of people who are there to help you so that you do not make the wrong choice and potentially lose all of the things you have been working so hard to gain throughout your life.

Just like our parents teaching us to say, "please and thank you," Tom Patire's program helped find that middle ground that my training was lacking by teaching the right things to say to get attention. In his book, *Tom Patire's Personal Protection Handbook*, which I think every household should have, he comes up with the best scripts for kids to say and adults to say to help get them out of bad situations. For example, kids in the age range of four to nine years old, in order to attract the attention of every responsible adult around them, should loudly say, "Stop touching me there!" Adults, in turn, will react immediately to see if it is appropriate or inappropriate touching. The script changes for older kids in middle school and high school. The red flag for teachers to immediately respond and help kids that are being picked on is the word *STOP!* followed by whatever is happening to the child at that moment. For example, "Stop hurting me, stop calling me names, stop teasing me, stop making fun of my family, etc." Teachers and parents can help students that are having problems come up with appropriate scripts that are specific to their situation.

For adults, the script changes, as most people do not get involved out of fear. Tom Patire explains that the best way for an adult to attract attention, whether you have kids or not, is by injecting a child's safety as the problem. A lot of people are told that yelling

"Fire" or "911" or "Help" are the best things to say to attract attention for help. If you yell "Fire" in a public setting, most people are compelled to evacuate the premises, because that is what we are conditioned to do. When you yell, "911, Help," some people, out of fear of getting hurt, will not want to get involved, or will assume someone else will make the call. If an adult yells, "Somebody help, they are hurting/taking my child!" whether they have a child or not, more people are willing to help, because they are coming to the aid of a child rather than to the aid of a male or female adult.

What script can a teacher or parent use to help break the cycle of bullying? Teachers struggle with knowing how to convey the message to their students on why they need to stop their abusive behavior. It is obvious through the media and internet that there is a nationwide problem with bullying in our schools. There are many different types of bully prevention programs out there, but yet, the problem still seems to be out of control. There seems to be a disconnect in communication between the teachers, parents, and students. In order for me to help relay my message of what scripts the teachers and parents can use, I share the stories from my friends in law enforcement about traffic stops. Police officers have to treat every traffic stop as a potentially life-threatening event, not knowing who they have pulled over and how they may react to being stopped. Most people, when they get pulled over by a police officer, are frustrated, get angry, and argue, saying, "There are other crimes being committed, why are you wasting your time pulling me over?" Police officers try to convey the message that, for every accident due to drunk driving, speeding, or text messaging, they are the first responders that show up to the scene. The officer sees fatalities of men, women, and children that the driver being pulled over cannot imagine. When issuing traffic tickets, the officer is doing his job by keeping the roads safe on his watch. It seems like a punishment to the driver, but it is really a step towards saving their life.

My message for parents and teachers when addressing the topic of bullying is to share their personal experiences from the past with the class. They need to tell the children, "I am approachable. If you are going through rough times, I realize the bully might say things to you to keep you from talking to me, other school staff members, or to your parents, but we can't help you if we don't know what is going on. We are all here to help keep you safe. I have dealt with bullying in the past, and have even had candlelight vigils for students who have committed suicide due to bullying, and I don't want that to happen again. Not on my watch." The teacher needs to show the students they genuinely care by sharing their experiences from the past. It may be a story from a previous experience as a teacher, or an experience they had as a child. They should let the kids know, for example, "When I was your age, I was bullied myself. As an adult looking back, this is how I wish I would have handled it." Then kids understand they are not alone, there are others who have been through similar experiences that know what they are going through.

I have found that there are many children and adults that do not know what to say because they have never been taught this as a part of learning responsibility. Once you know how to use the script to get help, you show responsibility by attracting the attention of safe adults, which will, in turn, enable you to get to a safe place. Families can train and practice their scripts in a creative manner by playing a game of "what would you do?" or "what would you say if…?" The parent may ask their child, "What would you say if someone asks you if you want to go for a ride in their car?" Or, "What would you say if someone asks you if you want to try a new drink or candy that makes you feel good?" What kind of script would you give your younger child to bring your attention to the situation? The best script that I have found for young children is, "I have to ask my parents." We all teach our kids to say "No" to strangers. This never brings our attention to who that stranger is and enables the stranger to go to another child, and another child, and another child, until eventually the untrained child will say "Yes." If your child's script was, "I have to ask my mom or dad," that in turn brings to your attention who is asking your child inappropriate questions so that you can protect your child and get a good look at the stranger or Wolf and their vehicle. Then, if anything bad happens to a child in your neighborhood, being the responsible adult, or Watchdog, you have a suspect or person of interest you can then turn in to the Sheepdogs. As parents come up with many different scenarios to test their kids on how they would react, it also helps reinforce those same skills for them as adults. Have you as a parent/teacher done everything you can to prepare them for living a life on their own?

Step Five —Find Safe People and Safe Places

Step Five means getting yourself back to the herd, and closer to safe people in safe places. A bully will try to isolate you in the bathroom or a remote corner of the school or parking lot. A criminal will try to force you into their vehicle, or pull you into their hotel room, into the bushes, or behind the dumpster. They want to get you alone, to make sure there are no witnesses to see the bad things that they have intended for you. It is important that you deny the bully or the criminal privacy by dropping your body weight and latching on to any objects around (a tree, a street sign, a door jamb, a fire hydrant, a bicycle). Hold on to anything that will slow the process down and buy you time while you are screaming your Script for Safety to attract attention. Do not let them take you to a secluded, private location where there is no one else around.

You need to get out of there and back to where other people are, where they can see and hear what is happening to you; and hopefully, among the herd, there is a Sheepdog or Watchdog that is willing to become a hero and take action. If, in the herd, no one is willing to take action to help after hearing your scripts or cries for help, there is a disconnect and a problem with society, and you will have to resort to *justifiable tactics in accordance with the law* to ensure your safety or the safety of loved ones. These tactics need to be learned from a professional, whose expertise focuses on reality-based training for personal protection, which is beyond the scope of this book. Any techniques learned need to be practiced correctly until they become a part of your lifestyle.

An example of finding a safe place can be seen when dealing with road rage. I may have accidentally cut someone off, then the aggressive driver lays on the horn and tells me "Pull over, *[expletive]*." Do I pull over in an isolated area? No! Do I go home? No! I go to a safe place like a mall, a police station, or a gas station where there is lots of lighting, possibly cameras, and there are many people who can see how out of control this person is and come to my aid.

To help parents, teachers, or yourself learn how to role-play to become assertive, below I have listed specific scenarios for kids, women, and men based on the most common situations they encounter at that stage in their life.

The most common scenarios for potential violence and bullying that I have come across include:

Kids' Situations	Women's Situations	Men's Situation
The bus stop	Abusive Relationships	Responsible father
On the bus	Sexual Harassment at work	The bully at work
In the school hallway	Sexual Assault/Trauma	Ego + alcohol/drugs
In the classroom	Crime	Treatment of women
In the school bathroom	Entrepreneurial woman	Being a sports parent
In the lunchroom	Parenting, Single Parenting	Example to children
During PE or recess	Teen pregnancy/abortion	Pressure for success
Dealing with strangers	Domestic Violence	

What I do in my workshops is have my attendees pick a situation that they've either found themselves in, are afraid that they may one day find themselves in, or just plain want to be prepared for. Then we review the "how to be assertive" steps, and then we role-play the situation they decided upon.

Here are the steps on how to be assertive for review:

Step One: Maintain a Safe Zone

Step Two: Adopt a "Good Guy" Stance

Step Three: Stay in Control

Step Four: Know Your Script for Safety

Step Five: Deny Privacy and Find Safe People and Safe Places

Role Play the Scenario

I have chosen a few examples from each list above to show how to apply all of the steps for handling each situation assertively:

Kid's Role Play:

In the Lunchroom, where someone butts or jumps in front of you in the lunch line

✓ Step One, the safe zone, means to back up to a safe distance away from the bully that cut in line to avoid physical confrontation.

✓ For Step Two, a good guy stance is standing with your hands up and open, showing that you do not want to escalate the situation, but you are ready to protect yourself.

✓ Step Three is keeping your cool and not getting angry, but not letting the bully get away with it either.

✓ Step Four is using the Script of Safety, or proper language, to attract attention, such as "Stop butting in line!" in a firm, loud voice over and over again, like a broken record (or a CD that skips if you do not know what a record is).

✓ Step Five is attracting safe people, or Sheepdogs, to help diffuse the situation. The teacher, or first responder, hears the commotion and asks what is going on. Between you and, hopefully, other bystanders or Watchdogs that want to be a part of the solution, the bully will get put in their place to learn responsibility.

Here is a true story of a child with special needs who had emotional and behavioral problems that was bullied on the bus.

Bully, Victim, or Hero?

I was conducting a workshop at a school in the Special School District, a school for children with special needs. One of the kids in the classroom said that he was bullied all of the time on the bus. He said that when he was picked on, he would get mad and would literally explode in a violent manner, causing damage to the bus and scaring the other kids with varied special needs. Usually, following the school's safety protocol, the police would need to be called, with the child being handcuffed and escorted off school property. I asked the child to come to the front of the class so we could role-play his scenario out and look at the consequences based on his previous behavior and actions versus the results he would see by following my steps and guidelines.

To simulate a bus, I brought up four chairs and lined them up. The teacher acted as the bus driver. I placed one child behind the driver as a bystander. The child being bullied is behind him. The bully sits in the back of the bus. I instructed the child pretending to be the bully to start teasing their intended target. I then asked the target how he would normally respond. He replied, "I would swing my fist, hit the windows, tear the seats, scream my head off, use vulgar language, and threaten everyone around me." Then, we role-played the bus driver giving out the usual consequence: a bus write-up, a detention, an in-school suspension, or, worst-case, arrest by the police. The bystander did nothing but help aid in provoking the bully to continue harassing his target.

I explained to the class that the behavior of the bully and the intended target losing control can distract the bus driver and potentially cause an accident, which may harm the other kids riding the bus. Then I set up a role-play using my guidelines. I took the role of the Victim and had the kid bully me. While I am on the bus, I cannot move into a Safe Zone. I need to stay in my seat. The only thing I can do is to turn around and assume a good-guy stance with open hands in a non-threatening position and use my Script for Safety. Assuming that there is lots of noise on the bus from kids talking and yelling, plus the noise the bus makes itself, the driver may not hear me using my script of safety like, "Stop hurting me, stop touching me there, stop being mean to me." I then demonstrate how the bystander, instead of being part of the problem, can get the attention of the bus driver. Once the bus driver is alerted to the problem and safely stops the bus, he or she can inquire "What is going on?" without you, the intended target, looking like a tattletale or snitch. So, the target saves face in front of his or her peers. The bystander's answers the driver's question, and the bus driver can get confirmation from the other bystanders who can say what happened.

Once the bus driver figures out what really happened and understands who really caused the problem, they will do the write-up on the real bully, and the target will not get in trouble. I tried to get the child who originally asked the question to role-play the new method. After several failed attempts (he would always go back to his old behavior), he was finally able to successfully do the role-play from start to finish.

The following week, when I returned to the school for additional training, the teacher excitedly approached me and said, "You will not believe what happened. I will let the student who was bullied on the bus tell you." When the student came into the class, he too was very excited and had a smile from ear to ear. He walked right up to me and said, "Guess what?"

I replied, "What?"

He said, "I tried what you told me to do on the bus when the kid was picking on me, and it worked!" He was so happy that, for once, he did not get in trouble. The instigating bully did. The boy said he was going to use his Script for Safety all of the time. I told him I was happy to help and for him to keep practicing his scripts so he could stay out of trouble.

By following all of my steps, this child was able to learn that there are positive, healthy solutions that he is able to choose without looking weak or losing face in front of his peers. It totally boosted his self-confidence and he was then able to build on that in other areas of his life.

Another time, I was at a middle school working with a group of kids where one had aggressive behavioral problems and anger issues. He was one of those kids that always looked pissed off at the world. The teachers went above and beyond in their efforts to use my program with this boy; they even took it to the next level to help him.

Through working with the staff and students on extensive role-plays and written exercises, the child started coming around with a more positive outlook towards school and life in general. He was making changes in his life to better himself, but he was still friends with some neighborhood kids that were in gangs. One day, though, he was with these friends, in the wrong place at the wrong time, and was shot and killed by a stray bullet. The story is tragic but the lesson is powerful: in order to truly make a difference towards moving in a positive direction, it has to be a lifestyle change. Sometimes that means changing your friends. Sometimes that means parents need to be more involved in knowing who their children are hanging out with. The communication between both the parents and teachers needs to work together to aid in the growth of the child.

We as parents and teachers need to work with the kids at an early age to get them into the Hero mindset. This trains them early on to be mentors not tormentors. I was working with a group of third grade students, introducing them to my Heroes in Action program. The kids took to the program and loved playing the role of the Hero. I used scenarios like, "What if your parents were sick or unconscious? What if your teacher was? Who can you go to for help? Who is the safe adult?" I had the kids role-play as bystanders how to be a Hero for someone being bullied by another child. They all wanted to volunteer to be the Hero.

Two weeks after I was at the school working with these kids, I got a phone call from one of the teachers. She said, "You will not believe what the kids did at the school." I asked what happened. She told me that normally there is free time where the kids can choose to do any activity that they want like read books, play outside, etc.

She asked her kids what they would like to do. Their reply was that they wanted to be Heroes for the kindergartners and first graders by helping them with anything that was needed. The teacher said the kids came up with this idea all on their own. I was so proud of those kids.

As I thought about this group of older, third-grade kids who wanted to be Heroes or mentors to younger kids, I looked at how high school and college is a breeding ground for bullying and hazing type behaviors by the upperclassmen towards the freshmen or lowerclassmen of the school. Instead of juniors and seniors calling freshmen "Fresh Meat," they should act as mentors and show them the ropes for becoming a positive part of a school that they are proud to be at. There are some schools that have mentoring programs where teachers train upper-class students to become peer counselors for new students and to break down the barriers of cliques, which in turn helps reduce different types of bullying.

A school in my area has taken students from each area of interest (drama, cheerleading, chess, all team sports, band, etc) and has taught them to be peer counselors or mentors to work together to make other students feel that they can join any group without fear of being ridiculed or mocked. They are showing more of what the school has to offer for their growth and education versus downplaying some activities, where a child may feel if they participated in that, they may be made fun of.

Women's Role Play:

Being a Victim of Sexual Harassment at Work

First, define the level of harassment. Is the bad employee making inappropriate gestures, or are they using inappropriate language, text messages, emails, or personal notes? Are they physically groping you, or making you feel uncomfortable? Are they using this to control your advancement at work? Do you know your rights?

✓ Step One, get into a safe zone where they cannot touch you or get physical with you.

✓ For Step Two, take a good guy stance to form a protective barrier between you and the bad employee.

✓ Step Three means keeping your cool. Do not let him intimidate you and push your buttons so you lose control.

✓ Step Four is using your script. You cannot wait an hour later, a day later, or a week later to tell this to anyone, because it is your word against the bad employee's. Draw attention to the situation immediately. Here are some scripts you can use: "I do not appreciate that gesture! I do not like you making that kind of comment to me! This is an inappropriate note! I do not appreciate you grabbing my A**!!" or, the best one, "What you are doing is sexual harassment and you need to stop it right now!"

✓ Step Five is making sure other employees are witnesses to your incident by attracting attention. That way it is not your word against his if you choose to pursue legal action, which I always recommend you do to help change his behavior.

Sexual Assault

This is a true story that I saw on national TV on a talk show. It was about a girl who was in a sorority that was going to a fraternity party with some friends. As she was there, a guy that she did not know began hitting on her. She had shown no interest in this guy, but he was very persistent. Later the same guy approached her and apologized for being so forward and asked if she would like to go somewhere quiet to talk. She did not think anything bad would happen, so she agreed. He took her to a room that was dubbed, "The Mattress Room." The only thing in this room was a mattress. No sheets, no pillows, no real lights. He closed and locked the door and proceeded to rape her. On the other side of the door, there was a party with loud music, people yelling, screaming, dancing, drinking, and having a good time. No one could hear her screams of fear and cries for help. When he was finished with his sexual assault, the girl put her clothes together and tried to get her sorority friends to take her back to their dorm. They did not want to leave because they were having too much fun. She scraped up enough money from different people to get a taxi cab back to her dorm. She ended up dropping out of college because of the trauma, attempted suicide a few times, and was in and out of mental health institutions for dealing with this trauma until she had the strength to be able to go on national TV and share her story so that other girls would not have to go through her trauma.

Let's apply my guidelines to her scenario and see if it could have changed the outcome. The two major issues here were the girl did not stay with her friends, with the herd, and she put herself in a position where she could not deny him privacy. She screamed and fought, but no one could hear her because of the other outside distractions.

Be tuned in not tuned out to what is going on around you. Always stay with the herd, and always deny the bad guy privacy. Trust your gut instincts. Her case may or may not have involved alcohol, drugs, or the date-rape drug, but know that anything that impairs your judgment can put your safety and the safety of others at risk. Whenever you can, meet friends at a central location and try to drive together. If taking separate vehicles, follow each other to your destination instead of saying, "I will meet you there," where you run the risk of being isolated in a parking lot. This might sound extreme, but given the society that we live in, I recommend that the person who gets the closer parking spot should get out of their vehicle and into the vehicle of their friends, who then find a further parking spot. They all walk in together as a herd, and they all leave together to the closer parking spot where they all then drive to the farther parking spots and follow each other out.

Sometimes we have to take more precautions to ensure the safety of ourselves, our friends, and loved ones.

Men's Role Play:

Being a Responsible Father

In each scenario, the five steps can be adapted to fit the circumstances. The following example will demonstrate how you adapt each of the five steps to a positive situation.

✓ Step One, the safe zone, can mean that I supervise my child and let them know that I am there for them to feel safe.

✓ For Step Two, a good guy stance is showing love, affection, and caring versus making a fist, using threatening body language, and being abusive.

✓ Step Three means teaching your child their responsibilities without losing control, and following through with age-appropriate consequences.

✓ Step Four is using the proper language to build your child's self-esteem, instead of simply yelling and cussing.

✓ Step Five is not bringing friends into your home that would be a bad influence or role models for your child, and not taking them to things like a Rated "R" movie that expose them to inappropriate situations.

Domestic Violence

Domestic violence could be a relationship between a boyfriend and girlfriend, husband and wife, or parent and child. How the parties involved in domestic violence will handle the problem in a healthy manner is determined by the environment that they surround themselves in, and whether they are willing to have a third party mediator or referee to help them open a line of communication. This mediator can be family, a friend of the family, neighbor, pastor, social worker, or in worst-case situations, the police.

I have worked with men that have been incarcerated for spousal abuse, most of which most were arrested for violence towards their spouse due to a drug or alcohol problem. These men did not look at getting into a safe zone, did not take a neutral, non-offensive posture ("the good guy stance"), nor used a script to diffuse or de-escalate the situation due to the influence of the drug or alcohol that they were under. The drugs and alcohol hindered their ability to be rational. Most of them said that they would never call the police because of their prior record, and the police, upon showing up to the scene, would not objectively listen to both sides. Instead, in their mind, they thought the police would automatically assume the one with the prior offenses would be at fault.

My advice to anyone who is feeling they need to be violent is to first get into a safe zone by leaving the scene for a cooling off period, or by isolating themselves in a bathroom or bedroom, away from the other person. Then, call someone to help mediate, like their friend, neighbor, pastor, or, in worst-case situations, 911. If 911 is called, your script to the operator can be "I've had a prior record for violence, and I am having an argument with my spouse, and I don't want it to get out of control. I need someone to help mediate this problem, so I don't do something that gets me back in jail. I just got a job, I just got a new house, etc., and I don't want to jeopardize that." I also encourage the spouse who has isolated him or herself to put the phone up to the door. Most likely the other spouse is yelling at and banging away, and the operator can hear the other party fueling the situation. When law enforcement arrives, they have this information and can be more objective in how they handle the situation.

Most of these men say that they wouldn't feel like a man if they were to call the police, but would feel like a pansy (and that's the nice way to put it) because they are not handling the situation on their own. Most men who are prone to domestic violence believe they are the "man" putting "their woman" in her place. My response to these men is to ask them if they enjoy the freedoms they have now while on parole. The freedom to spend time with their kids. The freedom to try to start a career and become successful at something in their life. The freedom to see friends, family, go on vacations, and enjoy holidays. Would they like all of those freedoms to be taken away because they'll be thrown back in jail as a repeat offender? Sometimes they give me the reply that "This is how I have been all of my life. This is who I am. I can't change. Take it or leave it!" There is no easy reply to someone with this thought process.

The only way that I have found I can make a connection is to get them to see things from a different perspective in comparison to themselves. I use the example of a person who enlists in the military who has been trained to kill the enemy. When a soldier spends hours upon hours of training and working as a team in a unit to go fight enemies, even looking at how long they stay in the military, and how much exposure they have had to war, still cannot allow you to predict the length of time that it will take for them to become re-acclimated for civilian life once out of the service. For a soldier, the effects of war, for instance taking a life for the first time, seeing a member of his unit lose their life, loss of hearing, sight, or limbs, or being captured by the enemy as a prisoner of war, makes it necessary for them to re-acclimate themselves to civilian life through extensive retraining, therapy, and counseling, which can take as little as a few months or the rest of their lives. I have personally worked with and seen soldiers that have gone to hell and back rebuilding their lives to get back to living happy, healthy civilian lives and work towards becoming successful. In my mind, if they can accomplish this, then any trauma or hardships anyone has gone through from childhood to present time can be overcome as well. I relate this back to my own personal story of how I have overcome my own demons from my past to become who I am today.

Most of these men, and sometimes women, do not have the script to know what to say in order to resolve common situations in relationships without resorting to aggressive behavior or violence. These situations can be blown out of proportion due to the influence of drugs or alcohol, friends, insecurities, pet peeves, financial situations, or illness. It is important to get the attention of healthy support groups around you to help you with your scripts and actions for making better choices in life, to not sabotage yourself, and possibly lose your freedoms.

Whatever the situation, I urge you to create role plays for each one using my equation listed above. In its simplicity, you need to be able to define the problem then use the equation to find the solution. Ask yourself, If I take a negative path, what will happen, what are the consequences? If I take a positive path, will the outcome change? What other factors can add to the problem? (For example, bystanders who will not be a part of the solution).

As I went through both stages of being passive and then aggressive, and finally getting to my new comfort zone of becoming assertive, I began feeling good about getting into a safe zone and using a script of safety without losing face in front of my peers. These steps taught me to progress from being the passive victim who was bullied in school and at home, to being the aggressive bully that did not want to be a victim anymore, to finally becoming assertive, finding that middle ground which has enabled me to achieve success without sabotaging myself.

I am proud of my accomplishments that I have achieved, but I did not get to where I am today without the help of family, friends, and people who believe in me. In order for people to believe in you, you have to be noticed in that positive light without sabotaging yourself, and not be afraid to ask for help. No Rambo's.

The Game of Life

I have been asked by teachers and parents, "What can we say to an aggressive person that is in our lives to help them make better choices?" For example, what could a teacher say to a student, or a parent say to a child, or a spouse say to an aggressive partner? I had to come up with an answer that everyone could relate to and understand, and apply it to every stage of life, from childhood to parenthood. I came up with what I call "The Game of Life."

Everyone can relate to sports that have tournament brackets, in which the final slot is your champion. Below is a graph of a tournament bracket that could be used for any sport, but for teaching purposes, I will use hockey.

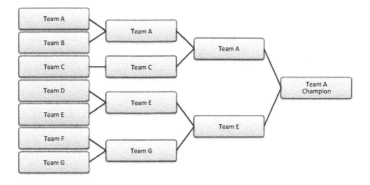

You have eight teams that are trying to compete for the number one spot, or the championship. In my lectures, I ask everyone attending how many of them want to be that champion in that final spot. Usually, 100 percent of the people attending the lecture will raise their hand, as they all want to be champions. Would you want to be that champion? Let's say that you are one of the key players on the team and, without you, it may affect the outcome of the game and whether your team wins or loses. Every sport has a referee that decides who wins or loses, and blows the whistle on personal fouls. You, the key member of the team, committed a foul and the referee blows the whistle on you and sends you to the penalty box for two minutes. As one of the key players, do you argue with the ref, or do you take the penalty? The people who are aggressive by nature may argue with the ref, which in turn, can get them kicked out of the game, costing the team the win to move forward and become the champions. I try to explain to aggressive individuals that, if they take the penalty and accept the consequence, they are able to stay in the game and their team can move forward towards the championship. My message is to take responsibility for your actions, and accept the consequences so you can stay in the game.

Below are examples of how this applies to every facet of your life. Start with your childhood:

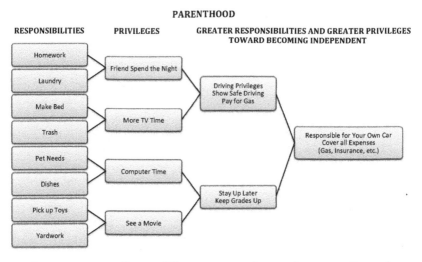

In every part of your life, you are going to have a referee that determines how fast you move forward towards reaching success. As a child, the referees at home are your parents or guardians. As a child, you have a goal of being a champion and to become independent. In order to reach this, you need to prove to your parents (the "referees") that you are responsible enough to go out on your own. Depending on your age, you have a list of age-appropriate chores (homework, laundry, etc). If you do what you are responsible for, you get privileges and get to advance forward. If you fail to do these, you get a "penalty" or lose privileges because you did not show you were capable or responsible.

As kids get older and demonstrate their ability to handle more responsibilities (driving a car, paying for gas, etc), they move closer to the championship position, or independence. For example, in our graph, independence is having their own car, which in turn gives them freedom to be less dependent on the parent to drive them around. As a minor, at any time, the referee can blow the whistle and send them to the penalty box. They will then have to earn back the respect and trust before they can move back to that level of independence.

The next stage is a child's education. Below is a graph depicting the progression of their education, of which the referees are the teachers and administrators who determine your advancement to the next grade level. The championship position is graduation. This graph is for graduating elementary school, then repeated for graduating middle school, then high school, and college or trade school.

EDUCATIONAL GRAPH TOWARD SUCCESS

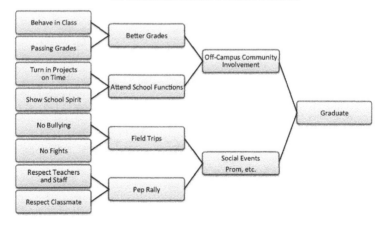

The graph shows the privileges students can receive as they make positive choices when moving towards the success of graduating. If they choose to cheat, fight, be disrespectful, skip school, or any other negative action, they will sabotage themselves by either being held back or expelled from school. For example, a student that cheats on a test and gets caught will get a non-passing grade, which can, in turn, hold them back, not to mention the embarrassment in front of other students. I made this mistake in middle school many times, which hurt my grades. A student who repeatedly fights gets sent to the principal, who in turn, based on the severity of his actions, may expel him.

As students, they have choices that can either earn them privileges and guide them towards graduating with success, or that can sabotage them into under-utilizing themselves (as my father would say) and limit their chances for success.

The next graph in the progression represents your career. Here I show how you can climb up the corporate ladder, with the championship position being the CEO. However, this graph can apply to any career path you choose, with the championship position being whatever your highest aspiration is.

CAREER GRAPH TOWARD SUCCESS

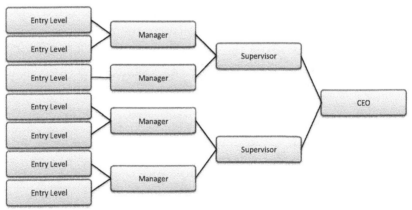

As you can see, you start with an entry-level position and work your way up to a management position, and eventually a supervisor position.

As a supervisor, if the CEO is looking for a successor to replace him/her upon retirement, if you know all of the ins-and-outs of the company, you will be the prime candidate. If you do not know the ins-and-outs of the company, and fail to advance through each position by not doing your job, then your "referee," or your boss, can pull a Donald Trump on you and say, "You're Fired!" As you become successful in your career path, then you can put more focus into other phases of your life such as relationships.

BUILDING SUCCESSFUL RELATIONSHIPS

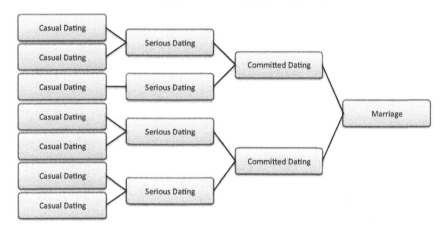

My dad had given me some of the best advice you could ask for in regards to relationships. He said, "Ray, date as many people as you can while you are young so you can figure out what you like and don't like." In this graph, I show the progression of casual dating as a way to figure out what you like and do not like based on who you are. If you are always looking at what you do not want or do not like, you are focused on the negative and will sabotage your chances of having a healthy friendship or relationship. If you focus on the positive and what you do want, you will have a happier, healthier friendship or relationship and can move forward towards the next level. In each stage leading to the championship spot, you and the person you are committed to are both referees in deciding the direction and success of the relationship.

Once you both have the commitment of marriage, you may decide that the next stage is planning to start your own family, or parenthood.

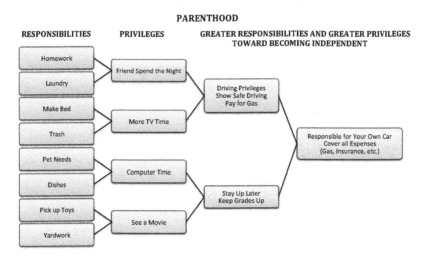

Once you are married and decide to have children, you become the referee as the parent, and the cycle starts all over again. You teach your child the responsibilities that you were taught by your parents as a rite of passageway to adulthood.

THE GAME OF LIFE

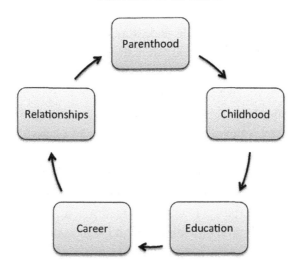

I call this "The Game of Life" because, from our childhood through our adult lives, we have referees in everything we do. By the choices we make, we have either negative consequences or positive outcomes. By illustrating with graphs and descriptions, my message to people who have a tendency to be aggressive or make wrong choices is to focus on being the champion and take the right steps necessary to move forward to reach the positive gains in life. Hence the phrases, "Did you bring your game? Is your game on? You've got game." If you go to jail, you lose your freedom and you are out of the game. My focus is helping you stay in the game and be successful in life.

9

Have You Sabotaged Yourself?

One of my first martial arts instructors, Mr. Fred Wren, told me a story a long time ago, when I first began competing in karate tournaments. The story had to do with fear and how it can either hurt you or help you. He said that, once he got into the black-belt division and starting making a name for himself, he was at a tournament and the first person he was chosen to compete against was the number-one ranked fighter in the country at that time. Mr. Wren said that he could have panicked at the thought of going up against this elite opponent. If he went in afraid, thinking that he could not win, then he would have defeated himself before even stepping into the ring. Mr. Wren, however, used his fear to his advantage. He stepped into the ring and, with great intensity, defeated his opponent. After the fight, this opponent came up to Mr. Wren and asked, "What got into you? I have never been beaten like that before." Mr. Wren's reply was, "I was so scared to get hit by you that I did not want to give you a chance to hit me." Mr. Wren took his fear and made it an advantage, rather than a disadvantage that could have cost him the championship. Now let's apply this to everything else in our lives.

Mr. Wren had shown me that it was his thought process first that affected his actions to get the outcome he envisioned. He showed me that, if my thought process is negative and I have a defeatist attitude, then my actions will be negative and I will not get the outcome that I wanted in the first place. If my thought process is positive, and I have the confidence that I can accomplish the task, then my actions that follow are positive, and I will be one step closer to accomplishing my goal.

I have seen many people, including myself, sabotage goals by starting out with the wrong thought process or attitude, brought on by low self–esteem, lack of confidence, and *fear*. Because I was not shown how to set goals and take the necessary steps to achieve them at a young age, I lacked the confidence to have a positive thought process to follow through.

When I was in school and still living with my mom and brothers, I would constantly be compared to my brothers and their better grades, my mother would belittle me, and the kids at school would bully me. Since I had no outlet, and no one to show me how to cope with what I was going through, I lacked courage, confidence, and self-esteem. My grades dropped, and I came to a point where I hated school and did not care. This was brought on by *fear*. I was afraid that I would never be good enough. I was constantly told that I was not good enough, and started to believe it. I began to sabotage myself because I did not care anymore. I stopped doing school projects, I did not turn in work, I cheated on exams, and I came up with excuses on why I could not finish homework. I lied. In my mind, if I was going to be a failure, I might as well act like one.

After I moved in with my dad and started taking martial arts lessons, my thought process changed. My dad's positive influence and guidance, combined with learning how to set goals through martial arts, gave me the courage, confidence, and self-esteem that I had lacked while living with my mom. In martial arts, I learned goal setting by going through all of the belt ranks, from white belt to black belt, which was a big confidence-booster. That training taught me how to set goals and accomplish them in all other areas of my life. I now felt that nothing could stop me from achieving what I wanted. My grades at school improved, my self-esteem grew, and I went from being an introverted, shy guy to being an extroverted, confident man.

I have seen people sabotage themselves with their family, friends, education, career, even their health. A lot of it is brought on by fear of not knowing what to say, of not knowing how to react, or fear of lacking the knowledge or ability to excel. They can sabotage their health and their relationships with the family through alcoholism, drug abuse, eating disorders, or by not properly addressing health issues that could be corrected through proper diet and exercise. They can sabotage a relationship with a spouse or a friendship by being dishonest, cheating, being violent, being financially irresponsible, or taking them for granted.

Peer influence, or feeling obligated to stand up for yourself or others, can be another form of self-sabotage. For instance, imagine you were standing next to your best friend and someone started talking about you, bullying you, provoking you, or pushing your buttons. Your friend might say, "Are you going to take that from him? Go take care of business. I've got your back!" Your good conscience might say, "Don't do it, get into a safe zone, look for ways to attract attention and stay out of trouble." Your bad conscience wants to impress your friend and not look weak in front of him, and wants to say, "Put this guy in his place, take care of business. Kick his @*#!" Most people I talk to in this scenario, especially kids in schools, listen to their bad conscience.

Let's go over what the consequences may be if I were to follow my bad conscience. I could go take care of business and hurt the person, maybe even permanently injure them or, worse case, because accidents do happen, I may take their life. I may win the fight, but I am the one responsible for my actions, and I am the one who has to take the consequences, even though it was my friend who talked me into taking care of business while he watched as a bystander. I sabotaged myself out of peer pressure and have to suffer the consequences. But it is not just me who suffers consequences. It is also my family. My parents will need to spend money for lawyers' fees to help defend me, which may have been my college fund. Depending on the severity of the lawsuit, they may lose other worldly possessions that are important to them. There may be a civil suit and a criminal suit, which could bankrupt them. If I am found guilty, I will serve time in prison.

By that same token, let's say my friend says, "Are you going to take that? Go take care of business. I've got your back!" As I confront the bully, I may not pay attention to my surroundings; maybe he has more friends that have his back, or he has a weapon like a knife or a gun. I become the one that gets injured, maybe permanently, or I am the one who loses my life, because my friend said, "I've got your back" but was not prepared for things to get that out of control. Now I suffer the consequences of being permanently injured for the rest of my life, or, worst case, losing my life, which will also affect my family. All of this happened because I was trying to impress my peers or not look weak in front of my peers. A true friend would have said, "We don't need to take this abuse from the bullies," whether the abuse is verbal or physical. The friend would have directed me to get into the safe zone and go to where there were more people and we had more options for creating a safe environment.

Let's take this situation. You are either standing with your mom, and someone is going off on her in front of you, cussing her out, saying vulgar, nasty things about her; or, you are at school, and someone is talking about your family, saying, "Your momma this, your momma that," and you feel the need to stand up for your family to defend their honor. I pose the question to kids and adults alike, "What would you do if someone was disrespecting your family in front of you?" The number one response I get is that they would fight that person, hurt that person, or beat up that person. They resort to animal instincts to protect their family, and immediately want to fight back. But, the same consequences apply as in the previous example, I hurt them or, worst case, take their life, I go to jail, my family has to pay the lawyers' fees, etc. Or, they hurt me and I am permanently damaged or worst case, they take my life, and my family has lost a loved one.

Another illustration of how making the wrong choice can sabotage you was the story of the "Hockey Dad," Thomas Junta, who killed his son's hockey coach, Michael Costin. This case drew national attention to the issue of parental violence at their children's sporting events. Junta did not like the way Costin was handling his son's game. Both of them got into a heated argument that escalated to a physical fight in front of all of the kids. Junta claimed that he was reacting in self-defense, but the jury found him guilty of involuntary manslaughter. The consequence was 6-10 years of prison time. There is a bigger tragedy than just a man dying and another receiving a 6-10 year sentence. The consequences of his actions affected everyone else who witnessed this tragedy, also. The Junta family now has a father that cannot provide for his family and who is missing out on the growth of his children during the stage where they learn responsibility and the rite to passage of adulthood, along with birthdays, school events, and holidays. The Costin family no longer has a father figure, and is constantly reminded of that on birthdays, school events, and holidays. All of the kids and parents at the game that day, along with the children of both families, will have to live with the trauma and image of someone's life being taken in front of them for the rest of their lives. Would you want your child to witness you getting injured or losing your life, or witness you injuring another or taking their life? Think twice, as you may not know what you are up against, whether it is in school, dealing with a childhood bully, or as an adult in a heated argument.

I am sure you could come up with many examples of how people can sabotage every area of their life. The main concept that we need to focus on is the initial thought process. I want you to pick up a pen or pencil and hold it up like I did when I started writing this book. You are now the author of your own story. At the end of each day, you choose what type of ending to write for that chapter. Do you want your ending to be a happy one or a sad one? Do not let others influence the outcome of your story. It is your thought process that enables you to choose how your day ends. It is taking your fears and deciding how you will let them lead you throughout each day. Are you afraid of relationships? Are you afraid of failing at work? Are you afraid of failing your family? It is your thought process, a positive outlook, and training that takes you to the level that enables you to follow through and accomplish your goals, so that, at the end of the day, you finish on a positive note.

As a part of my training, I learned to find out what signals my body sends me that causes the feeling of fear. Find out where fear hides in your body. Once you have found its hiding place, how do you control it and not let it overwhelm you? You are always looking for the signals your body sends you. Are your palms sweaty, your heart pounding, your face turning red, the veins in your head popping out, butterflies in your stomach, sweat beating on your forehead, the hair on the back of your neck going up, loss of bodily functions, your legs weak, shortness of breath? These are all signs that you are feeling fear. Instead of letting these feelings grow and take over your body, confront them, control them, and find ways to deal with them.

As discussed earlier, if you practice something twenty-five thousand times negatively, you will most likely have a negative outcome. If you practice something twenty-five thousand times positively, you will most likely have a positive result. It is the repetitive training with the positive mindset that enables someone to react without thinking and have the confidence to achieve his or her goals without fear. Mr. Wren trained extensively in order to be able to channel his fear to win his championship fight.

In order to not self-sabotage areas of your life, you must look at what you are afraid of within yourself and why you are afraid of it. Take this fear and channel it in a positive manner by getting the training that gives you confidence in yourself and keeps you from making bad choices.

10

It's a Lifestyle Change: Break the Cycle

If you were to take children ages one to two years old from every race, religion, and culture and place them together in a playpen, would they look at each other with prejudice? Would they refuse to play with each other because they look different? At what age does a child start looking at other people differently? What makes them change?

We are all products of our environment. Whether it is the way our parents have raised us, or the neighborhoods we have grown up in, or other outside influences, all of these are contributing factors towards how we view and react to others around us. The first man a newborn girl falls in love with is her father, and the first female she would want to be like when she grows up is her mother. The examples they set will affect her outlook on who she is and how she views other people when she gets older. The reverse would be true for a newborn boy and his parents. If a girl sees her father disrespecting the mother, degrading, belittling, and bossing her around, what type of relationships will she be likely to get into as she gets older, if this is all she has seen? If a girl sees her father being loving, caring, and respectful to the mother, and sees them resolve arguments and disagreements in a healthy manner, when she gets to the age of understanding and having relationships, she will compare any potential boyfriend who treats her badly to the positive way she viewed her father treating her mother. It is a clearer choice for her to leave an abusive or negative relationship based on the positive upbringing she had witnessed growing up as a child. In her mind, she will be saying, "My dad did not treat my mom this way, and I refuse to let anyone treat me this way!"

How many of you know somebody that always has that dark cloud following them? Everywhere they go, something bad happens to them. They are the biggest drama king or queen you have ever met. More bad things happen to them in a week's time than happen to you in a lifetime. You may even look at your life as boring compared to them. Is this drama self-sabotage? Does this stem from the ego's need for attention, regardless of whether it is good attention or bad attention? A student may get in trouble in school just to be the center of attention in the classroom. Another student may have to deal with rumor-spreading of he said/she said ("He told everyone on Facebook he would break up with me before telling me. I don't know how I can go on living!").

Both of these examples show the consequences of negative choices, where the people involved wanted to give up instead of realizing that they were young and they had plenty of time to learn how to look at things in a more positive manner and make better choices, as explained in the Game of Life. Then there is the paranoid adult in the bar who thinks everyone is looking at him funny, and gets into fights every time he goes out. He feels insecure and uses violence as a defense to prove his worth to others. People try different personalities to get a specific outcome. They may be funny, then cry, then be mean to get what they want. They keep trying until something works.

Below is a list of unhealthy personalities that people may adopt for dealing with fear, anger, or conflict. Do you fit into any of these categories?

1. **Tough Guy:** Someone who acts tough so people will be afraid of them and leave them alone.
2. **Trouble Maker:** Someone who looks sweet but tells lies to get what he wants and never gets caught.
3. **Loner:** Someone who likes to hide in her room and listen to music.
4. **Sleeper:** Someone who loves to sleep and forget anyone made him angry.

5. **Crier**: Someone who cries and feels helpless and that no one understands.
6. **Runner**: Someone who, when they are mad, runs away and says, "I don't have to take this."
7. **Silence**: Someone who shuts out everyone with silence as payback.
8. **Revenge**: Someone who says, "You are going to be sorry and I am going to get even!"
9. **Peace Maker**: Someone who may be mad but tries to make things okay and swallows their feelings.
10. **Hopelessness**: Someone who does not feel understood, and feels he has not received what is due to him in life and does not care anymore.
11. **Being different**: Someone who never feels like she fits in, takes the "Heck with them" attitude, and decides to be totally different and unique.
12. **Temper Tantrums**: Someone who makes a scene and continues the argument until he gets his way.
13. **Hitter**: Someone who feels she is entitled to hit because that is the way she was taught. "You hit me, so I can hit you back."
14. **Comedian**: Someone who uses sarcastic comments, keeps-em laughing, and then no one will ever know the difference.
15. **Sickly**: Someone who tends to have aches and pains when he is angry.
16. **Druggie**: Someone who uses pot, alcohol, or drugs to avoid the feelings of anger or pain.
17. **Dreamer**: Someone who pretends she is in a different world and takes revenge through her daydreams.

When kids would make fun of me, I would avoid eye contact, cry, freeze, run away, or try to take what they said and poke fun at myself. Like a class clown, I tried to be a comedian. After I began my martial arts training, I moved to the fight mentality, where I made eye contact, daring them to fight me. I would use sarcastic, smart-ass comments right back at them, challenging them to test me. It was like trying to heckle a comedian who would, in turn, verbally totally disable the heckler and make them look like an idiot. You cannot out-heckle a heckler. And I became a good one.

I am sure we can all list stories about ourselves or other people in our lives who, as products of their environment, keep making the same choices and the same mistakes without realizing that they have other options. That has been my problem since I was a kid growing up until early adulthood...I was not shown other resources that would give me options to make better choices. I had to go to the school of hard knocks and learn from my mistakes. If I had someone to show me how to be a better student and who made learning fun, then I would have felt more confident in myself in keeping up with my classmates in school. Instead, my mom yelled at me to read more books, and ridiculed me while comparing me to my brothers. I grew up hating school, hating to read, and always feeling I could never be as good as my brothers. Due to the lack of motivation to learn, and lack of confidence, I found I was sabotaging myself. I procrastinated on schoolwork, I was irresponsible with doing chores at home, and I isolated myself and became a loner. I wish someone had given me a list of places I could have gone to for help so I would not have to go through the school of hard knocks or live with the self-sabotage.

I come across a lot of parents that put their kids in as many different activities as possible, like soccer, swimming, baseball, gymnastics, dance, and karate so that their kids can find an interest or a hobby that they can get good at, which aids in building self-esteem. Not every family can afford to put their children into numerous activities so that they can experience and acquire social skills through these activities. So the problem is, what can parents who do not have the resources do to provide their kids with opportunities to excel in other areas other than just school?

Since I did not have a list of resources that could help me at my different stages in life, below I have put together a list of contacts that are meant to help people from early childhood through adulthood.

Early Childhood Resources:

* **Parents As Teachers**
  www.parentsasteachers.org

  This organization helps parents who are struggling with raising their newborn and young children.

* **National Child Abuse Hotline**
  www.childhelp.org

* **1-800-4-A-CHILD**

  This is a resource for children who have feelings of suicide and do not believe they have anywhere to turn for help.

* **Kumon**
  www.kumon.com

  This is a math and reading-tutoring program for children ages preschool through 12th grade, which helps kids build confidence and self-esteem in their abilities to improve their grades at school.

* **Sylvan Learning Centers**
  www.sylvanlearning.com

  This program tutors kids ages Pre K through twelfth grade, as an aide to help build confidence in a child's ability to finish schoolwork on an advanced level.

* **Boy Scouts of America**
  www.scouting.org

* **Girl Scouts of America**
  www.girlscouts.org

  These are value-based youth development organizations.

* **Boys and Girls Club of America**
  www.bgca.org

  This organization has trained youth development professionals that provide positive role models and mentors for children.

* Big Brothers and Big Sisters
  www.bbbs.org

  They provide successful mentoring relationships for all children who need and want them, contributing to brighter futures, better schools, and stronger communities for all.

Parents should always research their local chapters of these organizations for themselves, to make sure that their quality is consistent with their national standards for providing safe environments for children.

Young Adult Resources:

Below are organizations that are designed to get kids involved in programs that help build character, self-esteem, and a better value system as they move towards adulthood.

* YMCA
  www.ymca.net

* Local Church Youth Groups

* Local Community Centers

* Area Community College continuing education programs

* After-school programs

* Volunteer work for the elderly, the disabled, or people with special needs

Parents should always research their local chapters of these organizations for themselves, to make sure that their quality is consistent with their national standards for providing safe environments for children.

Adult Resources:

These resources are to help break cycles of behavior that negatively affect your personal lifestyle, your family, your work, or your career as an adult.

* Alcoholics Anonymous
  www.aa.org

* Narconon
  www.narconon.org

* National Domestic Violence Hot Line
  www.thehotline.org
  1-800-799-SAFE

* Suicide Prevention Hotline
  www.suicidepreventionlifeline.org
  1-800-273-TALK

* Narcotics Anonymous
  www.na.org

* Mental Health Network
  www.mentalhelp.net

* Gamblers Anonymous
  www.gamblersanonymous.org

* Eating Disorders Anonymous
  www.eatingdisordersanonymous.org

* Check your local hospital for specific group counseling

If I go back to my "What kind of a person am I?" list and find the answers with low scores that are in need of change toward a more positive direction, then I can focus on breaking some of my negative cycles and move forward in my Game of Life. We must all not be afraid to ask for help in breaking these self-sabotaging cycles we keep repeating.

Forgiveness

I have found that in order for me to truly move forward in life and achieve success, I have to learn from my past and not live in it. You can never forget the past, and should not let the bad events from it control you and possibly trigger your self-sabotage cycle. For me to do this, I have to forgive the people that have hurt me, and ask for forgiveness from the people that I have knowingly or unknowingly hurt. I was the black sheep of my family, but I was still a Sheep—still a victim. I turned into the Wolf for awhile, but now I am the Watchdog, the Sheepdog, the protector.

The most important person to begin forgiveness with is myself, knowing that I am not perfect, I am human, and I make mistakes. The things that I have done wrong in my past cannot be changed. All I can do is look at who I am now, and who I want to be, and make sure that I make those positive choices that enable me to move forward towards becoming that champion in the Game of Life, instead of holding myself back through self-sabotage.

I have to ask for forgiveness from my family. First, from my dad, for being the difficult son that challenged his authority instead of being grateful for his guidance, because I was tired of being told what to do and who to be. I neglected his insight as a parent showing me the passageway to becoming an adult. I did not give him a chance to be my dad. Please forgive me, Dad.

Next are my brothers, where my ego affected our relationship when we were young, due to envy. When I moved in with my dad, I pretty much cut off all contact with them, as I felt we had resentment towards each other when I left my mom. We all missed out on many years of birthdays, graduations, and family vacations, where I excluded myself from them. If you were to ask, "What kind of a brother was I back then?" I have to admit, I was not a good one, and that is why I ask for forgiveness. I realize that my brothers' hands were tied when they still lived with my mom, and it was not until they all went away to college, got married, and had lives of their own that we forgave each other for the things that happened in our childhood. My relationship with my brothers now is much better, but there is still room for improvement. We live thousands of miles apart from each other, which makes it difficult for us to grow as a family. But we will get there.

At the stage when I had transformed from the passive victim to the aggressive bully, I ask forgiveness from the people that I may have hurt or bullied along the way. I realize that my choices may have made them feel the same as I felt when I was bullied. I felt empowered by not being the victim any more. As I went from the one extreme of being the person who was controlled, to the other extreme of being the person who was in control, I let it get to my head. I saw who I had become, but it was too late for me to take anything back. For this, please forgive me.

For the bullies that tormented me in school, I forgive them for the verbal, physical, and emotional abuse that they had put me through. I no longer want to blame them for their behavior. I realize that they, too, lacked guidance and self-esteem, because they were products of the environment that they grew up in, just as I was. I wish them all success in life, and hope that they do not continue the cycle of abuse through their relationships.

Although my relationship with my mom is still not a very good one, I want to forgive her for the way I was raised when I lived with her. I realize that, coming from another country and culture, she had a limited education, limited social skills due to a language barrier, and no income other than alimony and child support from my dad. My mom was raising four kids the best way she knew how. She did not have the help of outside resources to give her guidance on how to be a better parent. According to my mom, it seems that her childhood, and the way that her parents had raised and treated her, was not that different from the way she treated my brothers and I. She did not realize the cycle that she was in, and was repeating her childhood through us, for that is all she knew. I hope that she also forgives me, as I know it is difficult to have a son leave you without knowing all of the reasons why. I did not just move in with my dad to get away from her. It was to get away from the school bullies and the environment that I was surrounded by, which may have led to a decision to commit suicide. I left because I wanted to live.

I would like to have a loving, caring relationship with my mom, but it is difficult as she always continues to live in the past, which she has a hard time letting go of. It is challenging having a healthy relationship when the history of her parents and family, her marriage and divorce from my father, and me leaving her always comes up. My hope for her is that she can find her own forgiveness for the people in her life and for herself. It is getting out of the victim mindset and taking responsibility for her own path towards happiness that will enable her to have loving relationships with her family and others.

I am able to forgive because I am happy with the man I have become. If it was not for the way I was raised and the experiences I had with bullies and relationships, I would not have sought out and been transformed by my martial arts mentors. They enabled me to put the pieces together for which I have chosen to make my life's mission, which is helping others help themselves.

For those of you reading this book, I hope you realize that this chapter helps you understand what kind of a person you are. It is your choice to forgive or not to forgive. If you choose not to forgive, you will sabotage every area that we have discussed in previous chapters. I ask again, why are you here? If you hang on to anger and issues from the past, it is hard to move forward. Who are you? What kind of a person are you? Are you the kind of person that will not forgive? Do you care? If you do not care, it leads to repeating the same cycles and sabotaging events and relationships in your life. If you do not forgive, you cannot make lifestyle changes for a better future, because you are stuck in the past. Learning to forgive can be difficult, but it is necessary if you want to be someone that has the power to help yourself.

12

Live Like a Hero

At the end of any class, lecture or seminar, I always ask everyone this last question…"What have you learned?" You can review your notes on who you are or what kind of a person you are, and rewrite them as often as you like to gage how far you have come at improving your quality of life. How many of your strengths did you make stronger? Did you improve any of your weak areas and turn them into strengths?

I have come up with a simple way to keep myself in check. It is three simple goals.

Goal #1: Train Like a Champion. A champion or winner of any sport puts a lot of time and effort into preparing to become that elite athlete. You must put as much time and effort into everything that you do with your faith, family, education, and career, so you can strive to become a champion in all areas of life. It is not about winning a trophy, which, over time, just becomes a dust-collector. The true trophy is that feeling inside that you get with a sense of accomplishment and pride.

Goal #2: Respect Your Body. You are sabotaging yourself by not eating healthy and exercising. I know this because I abused my body with a poor diet and alcohol for a long time. The injuries that I have sustained from over-training, or being too extreme, have taken a toll on my body as well. You need to take care of your body in order for you to continually be able to provide for yourself and your family. As we live in the world of "now" (i.e. fast food, fast internet, microwaves, etc), where we are trained to be impatient, it is healthy to give yourself more time to rest. There were times that I would work sixty to eighty hour weeks, running my own business, which in turn sabotaged my time with family, friends, and myself. You are disrespecting yourself if you abuse your body physically and sexually in ways that affect relationships with friends or family.

Goals #1 and #2 involve wanting the best for yourself, and taking the time to be healthy so that you are able to be selfless in your actions towards others in your life. Without doing goals #1 and #2, it makes it more challenging to accomplish your third and final goal.

Goal #3: Live Like A Hero. Living like a hero is not about you, but it is about what you do for other people. You try to take some time every day to do one selfless act for someone else. If everyone were to focus on helping others, not for personal gains but for doing the right thing, there would be less crime and suffering in our communities. Being a hero requires what I call the Three C's: Common sense for making better choices; Caring, which is going out of your way to help someone; and Courtesy, or being respectful to all those around you.

If, after reading this book, you walk away learning just one thing, I have done my job. If I have provoked thought, whether you agree or disagree with me, as long as I get you to research and find the answers you are looking for, I have done my job. My hope is that this book has given you insight into yourself so that you do not have the victim or bully mindset, but rather the hero thought process, where you rise from rock bottom to being at the top of your game of life.

Epilogue

The following pages contain two poems I have written over the years that share the content of all of the previous chapters in this book. I thought it would be a peaceful way to end this book on being assertive, for that is the whole point: to find peace in yourself and create peace in your surroundings. I hope you enjoy them.

Respect For Life

I've got four basic rules to follow by,
These rules, when applied, might save your life.
The rapes, the gangs, the killings
Will it ever end?
Has it come to teaching violence
To survive and defend.
The first rule, hey, is avoid and ignore
Instead of just fighting, let's learn and explore.
The second rule is talk
Hey, let's talk it out
There's no need to fight,
There's no need to shout.
Don't use words of aggression or words of plea,
Stand up for yourself assertively.
The rapes, the gangs, the killings,
Will it ever end?
The drugs our kids are selling,
Instead of making friends.
Don't just stand around in silence and watch in vain
Draw attention to what's happening and help stop the pain.
Don't forget to speak while you turn the other cheek
Use your words to let them know that you're not really weak.
I'll break it down to you, some advice for free,
Get a support group is rule number three.
Yeah, you can make it work, if you try you'll succeed
Just have your family, your friends and school by your side,
And help stop the violence
So you can live with pride.
Now learn to survive, that's rule number four
It's about getting away, not staying to play
So you don't wind up hurt or dead on the floor.
Don't stand around, don't wait for more
Just hurt and run, Hey that's rule four.

Epilogue

I pray and plead rule four is not needed
Use rules one through three and you'll never be defeated.
Don't be a part of the problem, be a part of the cure
Help stop the violence so you can live your life pure.
You've got to show some respect, respect for life
Gotta put down that gun and get rid of the knife.
We gotta be willing to stop all the killing
And show some respect, respect for life
I said! Show some respect, respect for life!

Heroes In Action

There was a small child
Whose imagination would run wild.
His favorite toy was a superhero
He wanted to become that toy, and dreamt that he was that hero.
He wanted to be a Hero In Action
Where he was fighting for what's right
And defending against what's wrong
That's right, a Hero In Action.
As he was growing up, he was bullied by some kids.
He didn't know what to do
And felt he had no one to turn to.
He didn't want to fight
'Cause he didn't feel that it was right.
So he started learning self-defense
And what he learned was common sense.
And he became a Hero In Action.
He was fighting for what's right
And defending against what's wrong.
He became a Hero In Action.
He was taught to turn the other cheek
But that only made him feel real weak.
He wanted to stand his ground
And have the bullies all back down.
'Cause if you let them get away with it,
They'll come back and have their way with it.
So he learned to use his words
To get attention to the herds.
The solution that he'd found
Wasn't fighting, but to get more people to stand their ground
And become
Heroes In Action where we are all
Fighting for what's right and
Defending against what's wrong.

'Cause you know the moral of this song
Is to get everyone to get along.
We can work together to find the peace
And rid the violence in our streets.
The answer is in front of us
Don't ignore it as it creeps up on us.
Don't come up with more resolutions
Just take action and be a part of the solution.
Don't just stand around and think, "What the heck?"
Use your words and actions
To be Heroes that are meant to serve and protect.
So we can all be!
Heroes In Action,
Where we're fighting for what's right
And defending against what's wrong.
We ARE Heroes In Action!

Appendix A

Recap of Helpful Rules and Tips

Below is a recap of five simple rules for kids in school to follow without fighting to not be victims of bullying or violence at school, as most schools are fight-free or zero-tolerance schools.

1. **Personal Space:** Stay in a safe zone, do not get into a danger zone.
2. **Body Language:** Be a good guy, keeping your hands open, and not aggressive, vs. the bad guy, balling up your fists where you may be perceived as the aggressor.
3. **Script of Safety:** Uses a specific script to attract attention for self-advocacy or to be a Good Samaritan helping someone who cannot help themselves.
4. **Safe Adults:** Learn to identify "good" and "bad" adults, and make the choice that gives you the positive outcome.
5. **Safe Area:** There is safety in numbers, so always run to the crowd and have an exit strategy where you have pre-determined safe places to go to.

This next list is for your personal safety, as a child or an adult. This list encompasses everything discussed in this book.

Ray's Top Ten Safety Tips

1. Don't think like a victim.
2. Know your safe zone.
3. Scan your surroundings for: Exits, potential threats, bystanders and objects that can be used as survival tools to get to safety.
4. Have a verbal plan or "Script of Safety." Draw as much attention to yourself as you can.
5. Deny the bad guy privacy.
    Drop your body weight and latch on to large objects like a street sign, a tree, or a door jamb to make it difficult for the "bad guy" to take you to a secluded location.

6. Know the weaknesses of the body and practice how to use specific movements to create windows of opportunity to escape.
7. Don't let yourself get distracted or suckered.
8. Always prepare and condition yourself mentally, physically and emotionally so you can overcome fear, panic, and hesitation in the event of any type of assault. (Practice, Practice, Practice—remember the rule of twenty-five thousand).
9. Share this information with loved ones, friends and co-workers to keep it fresh in your mind. Make this a routine part of your lifestyle, as it is a lifestyle change.
10. BE A HERO (Watchdog or Sheepdog) and don't let the bad guy get away with anything!

About the Author

Ray Amanat has dedicated his life to educating the public on personal safety and fitness.
His goal is to help everyone that seeks him out
for guidance, to learn how not to be a victim of
violence or become a victim of themselves. He
has his own unique way of teaching how to make
better choices in life with regards to health and
personal safety.

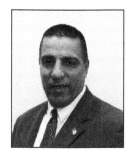

With over thirty years of Martial-Arts training and owning a
fitness and karate center since 1986, Mr. Amanat offers programs that
would get the whole family involved. Not everyone wants a Black Belt,
so Amanat developed specific programs that are reality-based and not
sports-oriented. "With sport martial arts, there are rules. When it comes
to survival and your life may be in jeopardy, there are no rules."

Amanat's goal is to teach a well-rounded program that would answer
the most common types of threats. He sought out experts in every
fighting style to be able to provide enough knowledge to his clients to
handle different levels of threats.

"I always ask people who inquire about my programs if they would
be prepared for any of the following types of threats: Are you physically
and mentally prepared for someone who knows how to box? Someone
who knows how to kick? Someone who is a good grappler or wrestler?
What if they had an impact weapon like a baseball bat? Or maybe an
edged or bladed weapon? Finally, do you know what to do if they have
a firearm at close range or outside of arms reach? If you answer no to
any of these, then when do you want to start training?"

Amant has worked with a number of school districts in the St. Louis area, including the Special School District for children with special needs and Hazelwood school district, delivering a series of staff training for school counselors and school assemblies on child safety and bullying. He has also delivered seminars to the Missouri Middle School Association and the Character Education conferences.

Ray Amanat is available for lectures and hands-on seminars for child safety, bullying, women's safety, and personal protection for the independent adult. For more information on any of his programs, workshops, school lectures, and seminars, please contact (314) 570-0243.

Email: respectcenter@sbcglobal.net

Website: www.respectcenter.com

Website: www.amanatsheroesinaction.org